HOW TO BEGIN REFORMING THE MEDICAL CURRICULUM

An Invitational Conference
Sponsored by the Josiah Macy, Jr. Foundation
and Southern Illinois University School of Medicine

Edited by Howard S. Barrows and M. J. Peters

Southern Illinois University School of Medicine

HOW TO BEGIN REFORMING
THE MEDICAL CURRICULUM

An Invitational Conference
Sponsored by the Josiah Macy, Jr. Foundation
and
Southern Illinois University School of Medicine
June 14 - 15, 1984

Editors
Howard S. Barrows
M. J. Peters

Editorial Staff
John T. Bruer
Glen W. Davidson
Beth Dawson-Saunders
Linda H. Distlehorst
Paul J. Feltovich
Terrill A. Mast
Charles E. Osborne
Nu Viet Vu

Southern Illinois University School of Medicine
Springfield, Illinois

Library of Congress Catalog No: 84-51789   Published 1984
ISBN: 0-931369-00-2   Printed in the United States of America

Contents

Foreword

As the tenth commencement of Southern Illinois University School of Medicine was contemplated, many people associated with the institution felt that this milestone should be celebrated in conjunction with another event affirming the school's mission or philosophy. Since curricular design and educational scholarship have been recognized strengths of this medical school, an educationally-oriented event seemed both logical and desirable. The increasing national concern about curricular abuses suggested that a conference focusing on curricular reform issues would be appropriate, as well as timely. Discussions with representatives of the Josiah Macy, Jr. Foundation, who felt that such a colloquium would provide a unique and positive approach to these mounting concerns, resulted in the foundation's agreement to co-sponsor the conference. The planning, selection of participants and structuring of the general flow of events were the products of many discussions among John Bruer of the Macy Foundation and Richard Moy, Reed Williams, Carol Bressan, Linda Distlehorst and Howard S. Barrows of Southern Illinois University.

The invited participants comprised two groups: educators and teachers actively involved in curricular innovation, and deans and senior faculty from a geographically wide range of long-standing traditional medical schools who recognize that there are problems with current medical education practices and who face the difficult task of implementing curricular change. It was hoped that these participants would create a unique working group, blending educational inventiveness with long practical experience in institutional change.

To stimulate interchange among the participants, the educators and teachers were asked to prepare preliminary papers addressing the question of how curricular reform might be undertaken. These "protagonist papers" were then circulated to those in the second group, who were asked to respond to the ideas presented and to provide additional commentary on any of the curricular reform issues they wished to address. The result of these efforts was a valuable and expansive collection of papers which provided the themes on which the conference agenda was based. The protagonist and response papers are included as Appendixes A and B.

One editor (HSB) served as moderator for the entire conference, while the other members of the editorial staff monitored the discussions as recorders. Although all recorders took notes throughout the two-day event, the responsibility for detailed, almost verbatim notes was rotated among pairs of observers in two-hour blocks. To prevent interruption of the flow of the discussions, no tape recordings or stenographers were used.

In the days immediately following the conference, the editorial group—with the great flexibility of a word processor and the assistance of a skilled operator, Bonnie Murphy—reconstructed what had been said to create a distillation of the colloquium. The ideas expressed in the proceedings are usually those of individual participants; in no way is consensus by the group implied. For the sake of clarity, consensus statements are presented separately. Individual names are purposely omitted from the ideas presented here, since the discussions were often very open and frank. Thus, the reader is allowed to gain important insights and to be privy to discussions that otherwise might never appear in print. Finally, a concerted attempt was made to keep these written proceedings brief and concise. They describe the flow and sequence of ideas as they occurred. Several key points which were repeated at various times during the conference are repeated here. No attempt was made to organize the ideas or topics in any formal way.

Although many people contributed to the success of this conference and devoted many days to it, both before and after, special thanks must be given to Linda Distlehorst, who with great skill, patience and endless hours of work engineered all the forces, people and events that led to what in many eyes was a flawless and highly productive conference.

Participants

Stephen Abrahamson, Ph.D.
Chairman
Department of Medical Education
University of Southern California

Howard S. Barrows, M.D.
Associate Dean for Educational Affairs
Professor of Medicine and Medical
   Education
Southern Illinois University
School of Medicine

Richard E. Behrman, M.D.
Dean
Case Western Reserve University
School of Medicine

Arnold L. Brown, M.D.
Dean
University of Wisconsin
Medical School

John T. Bruer, Ph.D.
Program Officer
Josiah Macy, Jr. Foundation

William Dignam, M.D.
Professor of Obstetrics and Gynecology
University of California, Los Angeles
School of Medicine

James B. Erdmann, Ph.D.
Director, Division of Educational
   Measurement and Research
Association of American Medical
   Colleges

Charles P. Gibbs, M.D.
Assistant Dean for Curriculum
University of Florida
College of Medicine

Marilyn Heins, M.D.
Vice Dean
University of Arizona
College of Medicine

James G. Hirsch, M.D.
President
Josiah Macy, Jr. Foundation

Gordon T. Moore, M.D.
Director, New Pathway Project in
   General Medical Education
Harvard Medical School

Richard H. Moy, M.D.
Dean and Provost
Southern Illinois University
School of Medicine

Vic R. Neufeld, M.D.
Chairman, M.D. Program
McMaster University

Lloyd H. Ramsey, M.D.
Associate Dean
Vanderbilt University
School of Medicine

Frederick C. Robbins, M.D.
President
Institute of Medicine

Consensus Statements

1. Reform is urgently needed; today's undergraduate medical students will be entering practice ten years from now. The tasks facing graduates ten to twenty years from now will be so complex, difficult and different that this is sufficient reason for every medical school to seriously consider curricular reform.

2. In its redesign of accreditation standards for the medical education programs leading to the M.D. degree, the Liaison Committee for Medical Education (LCME) should require each medical school to have commencement objectives* that include attributes of clinical performance. Furthermore, schools should be required to demonstrate that they use evaluation procedures which can measure these objectives.

3. Numerical scores on the Part I examinations of the National Board of Medical Examiners (NBME), as they now exist, are insufficient in themselves for the selection of applicants to graduate medical education programs.

4. The Medical College Admissions Test (MCAT) should not be used as the sole basis for excluding someone from consideration for admission to medical school.

5. The evaluation of medical students for promotion and progress must include examinations that assess more than cognitive skills such as memorization, recognition and recall of facts and concepts.

---

* Specifications of the competencies and abilities expected of students prior to graduation.

The Moderator's Charge to the Participants Based on the Ideas Expressed in Their Papers*

"No human arrangements are free from faults. A strenuous effort to improve and render perfect what already exists constitutes the task of life. Where can such endeavors be more justified or demanded than in dealing with the education of doctors on whose knowledge and ability the health and lives of men are so greatly dependent?"

—Theodor Puschmann, 1891
A History of Medical Education
(facsimile edition — New York: Hafner, 1966)

The exchange of papers among participants has identified a wide range of problems and approaches. The papers both reinforce and complement each other in very instructive ways. Each participant has had an opportunity to express his or her individual ideas and concerns and to see how these match with those of other participants. I have attempted to synthesize this opera into ideas that suggest the agenda for the conference.

There Is a General Consensus on the Kinds of Curricular Reformation That Should Occur

The papers of the participants and the many other recent writings about the problems of medical education all seem to agree on teaching practices that should be minimized and those that should be stressed.

---

* This statement by Dr. Barrows was sent to the participants with the agenda for the conference prior to their coming to Springfield.

1

Teaching practices that should be minimized:

- Content overload
- Stress on minutae not relevant to the practice of medicine
- Passive learning, particularly in lectures
- Emphasis on memorization of facts
- Use of tests that stress memorization of facts

Curricular themes and practices that should be stressed:

- Problem-based learning
- Self-initiated learning
- Critical analysis of literature and other information resources
- Cost containment skills
- Health maintenance skills
- Disease prevention skills
- Use of tests that assess problem-solving and the application of information
- More accurate assessment of clinical competencies
- Recognition of faculty for quality and quantity of teaching
- Increased personal contact with students in small groups

There Is Nothing New Since '32!

Dr. Swanson submitted a series of quotations from a 1932 book, *The Report of the Commission on Medical Education.** The commission was chaired by A. Lawrence Lowell, President of Harvard University, and sponsored by the Association of American Medical Colleges (AAMC). These quotations raise the same issues about medical education that the participants and many others have voiced in recent years:

> The medical course, partly because of the requirements for licensure, has been concerned more with the factual matter a student has memorized at the time of graduation than with the development of intellectual resourcefulness and sound habits and methods of study. Too great an emphasis has been placed on description and the memorizing of many details and facts which, though they are of little permanent

---

* *Final Report of the Commission of Medical Education* (New York Office of the Director of Study, Association of American Medical Colleges, 1932).

significance, are of immediate value in passing the examinations and in meeting the requirements of licensure to practice.

Inasmuch as medical education is primarily concerned with the qualifications and preparation of students to practice medicine, it is highly important that the training be permeated with an understanding of the larger social and economic problems and trends with which medicine must deal, and which are likely to influence the form and opportunities of practice in the future.

The present system of detailed subject examinations, which rely so largely upon memory and which are still popular in secondary schools and some colleges, tends to defeat the major purposes of the training, which are not the collection of facts but the intelligent and discriminating use of knowledge which is applicable to a given problem.

Furthermore, many other dedicated teachers and medical educators have repeatedly articulated these same concerns in the fifty years since that report. The martyrs referred to in Dr. Abrahamson's paper must be among their ranks. Therefore, despite the fact that these same problems have been identified frequently in the past half century by prestigious panels, educators and teaching faculty, the advertised concerns and suggested changes of these groups obviously have had little impact. This is a clear message that more effective steps must be taken and more powerful moves must be intitiated to achieve curricular reform. If not, our present deliberations may suffer the same fate. What a waste of energy that would be!

What Is the Problem?

The previous lists of practices that should be minimized and those that should be stressed are prescriptions. They identify treatments without actually identifying the problems. Instead of prescribing treatments, it might be better to state the problems that have been caused by traditional medical education practices. Such a statement may make more apparent the need for reform and allow individual schools to correct the problems using methods best suited to their values and educational philosophies.

If we take the suggested prescriptions and convert them into the problems they seem to be addressing, the troublesome issues in medical education might be expressed like this: 1) Students graduating from medical school do not enjoy their experience in medical education. They feel it is an ordeal which one must survive in order to become a physician. 2) Students graduating from medical school are neither effective nor efficient in their problem-solving, clinical reasoning and decision-making skills. 3) Students do not keep up-to-date effectively, do not have good self-assessment skills to determine strengths and weaknesses in handling the problems they face daily, and are unable to correct those weaknesses through appropriate self-initiated continuing education. 4) Students are not proficient in health maintenance, disease prevention and cost containment skills. An additional implication in these educational prescriptions is that the educational programs in most medical schools are inefficient; a great deal of time is wasted on teaching and memorizing much that is not important to the profession of medicine. Many participants will want to add to, correct or modify these statements, but there is reasonable consensus that these are among the problems in medical education that necessitate curricular reform.

Strategies for Reform Internal to the Medical School

One group of proposed strategies for reforming the curriculum involves internal approaches that could be undertaken by individual medical schools. Some participants argued that leadership within the school, usually the dean or a cadre of educational leaders, is needed to present an authoritative voice which will provide the impetus for curricular reformation. Many of the suggested processes for initiating curricular reform involve the formation of task forces, retreats, special committees, curricular reviews, faculty-wide discussions and goal statements.

Several participants recommended changing the organization of the school to allow for a corporate responsibility for education. Additional suggestions included a variety of budget strategies to reinforce curricular reformation and educational effort.

Others encouraged the development of opportunities for faculty education and training. Over the years such opportunities have been offered by different schools around the country. However, it takes more than the existence of such educational opportunities to cause faculty to learn about education and to acquire new skills in teaching. By increasing the rewards for teaching, and especially rewards for educational scholarship, the use of such educational opportunities may be promoted.

A strategy set forth in many papers was to develop effective methods for faculty evaluation. Evaluation is necessary to reward educational scholarship and to stimulate ineffective or nonproductive faculty to change.

Both the University of New Mexico and Harvard are examples of traditional schools which have isolated a subpopulation of faculty and students to develop an innovative curriculum. The University of New Mexico has been doing this for a number of years, and Harvard's program seems to be under way. Both institutions have used external funds for this approach. Certainly, curricular reformation by such a prestigious medical school as Harvard should influence other schools to consider similar changes. However, some participants were skeptical about approaches using a subpopulation of students, citing such concerns as the Hawthorne effect, the need for continued financing, and the limited effect, if any, of the program on the entire school.

Many participants believed that internal approaches to reform of the curriculum might be destined for an uphill fight, as the forces resisting change in most medical schools are powerful. Medical schools have traditional rewards and paths of responsibility that work against corporate responsibility for education, as well as against the extra time and effort spent at curricular reformation. The faculty have to *want* change. This is difficult to accomplish, since many faculty do not perceive that there is a problem with the way they educate medical students. The students' scores on the examinations of the National Board of Medical Examiners (NBME) are satisfactory, and the faculty's real rewards come in research, resident teaching and remuneration for clinical services. Furthermore, several participants pointed out that completely innovative schools were never traditional to start with. It was necessary for traditional schools like Harvard and the University of New Mexico to isolate a subset of students and faculty to effect a reformation. The collected papers suggest that, unless increases in pay, promotion, and perquisites are attached to educational endeavors, these pursuits will not compete favorably with research and clinical service activities.

Finally, any change which depends on an individual or a group of individuals within the school is apt to be temporary or short-lived because these key people may move on to new positions or become fatigued with the effort. Thus, it would seem far more powerful to concentrate efforts on the external forces that will effect and maintain change.

Strategies for Reform External to the Medical School

The use of external forces to bring about a reformation of medical school curricula was suggested in a majority of papers. One suggested that a national teaching award be given by an organization such as the AAMC. Of course, the agency giving the award would have to establish the criteria for excellence and the mechanisms for evaluation of candidates. Increased funding for educational research was identified as one means to facilitate change and provide incentive and recognition for faculty concerned with education. Along this line, several participants raised the possibility of the funding of curricular innovation by private foundations or by the government. The federal government already has demonstrated its ability to influence medical education through financial and legislative incentives for developing family practice and primary care programs, increasing the number of medical schools and students, and promoting research through National Institutes of Health (NIH) funding. Government control is not always sensitive to individual need, however, and a federal prescription for curricular reformation might not be the most effective or most desirable solution.

Other external forces such as pressure from university presidents and from the public were also mentioned as possible ways of encouraging educational reformation. The challenge provided to faculty by President Derek C. Bok of Harvard in his 1982-1983 annual report to the Harvard Board of Overseers was cited as an example of such pressure. A concerted response by medical students—the actual consumers of the educational process—was also suggested.

Many participants argued that the AAMC, NBME, American Medical Association (AMA), and the Liaison Committee for Medical Education (LCME) might be engineered into positions that could have a lasting influence on medical education, since these organizations are all in a position to certify medical schools and medical students. Several papers advocated a change in the LCME standards for medical school accreditation as a way to achieve reformation. The tenth draft of the proposed, revised LCME guidelines contains many elements that could directly encourage curricular reformation. If these guidelines could be further modified and utilized for self-study and accreditation, a potent force for curricular revision might be realized.

The AAMC project on the *General Professional Education of the Physician* (GPEP) may also become a potent force for change. One writer suggested that this study might lead to "non-permission" for schools to maintain their status quo. Other external groups such as the National Residency Matching Program (NRMP) and state boards were mentioned as possible external influences for change.

Changing the Test May Solve Many Problems

One recurrent comment made by many participants was that, despite the advertised concerns of a handful of medical educators, most faculty do not truly believe that there is a problem with the present medical curriculum. No one is interested in fixing something that isn't broken. Faculty have a complacency, as pointed out by Dr. Abrahamson, that is one of the most powerful inhibitors of change.

Medical school faculty feel comfortable with their students' good NBME examination scores and with the performance of those select students that stay on in their residency programs. The faculty are convinced that they are doing a good job and no change is needed. They must see that there is a problem in their product before any meaningful changes will occur.

Probably the best way to allow faculty to see that there is a problem is to change the types of examinations used in medical schools from those that primarily stress recognition or memorization of facts to those that assess the behaviors and skills that we all believe are important in the physician. No one will ever know whether students have difficulties with problem-solving, patient evaluation, self-initiated study, health maintenance or disease prevention, unless these skills are assessed. It clearly is not enough for a student to be able to write down on a piece of paper what he or she would do in practice. These evaluation issues were addressed in various ways in the protagonist and reactor papers:

> "Few of us regard the NBME examinations or any other test to be adequate to define the physician we wish to produce."

> "How little of the goals described (Harvard, McMaster University of Mexico) is amenable to multiple choice questions, NBME, FLEX."

> "It would be helpful to join in discussions with an agency to accelerate development of evaluation tools which test important competencies, to minimize abuse of NBME examination results."

> "A review of the microbiology final exams of about two dozen medical schools and a subset of the NBME test item library of multiple choice questions leads to the conclusion that over 90% require only recognition of isolated facts."

American Psychologist recently published a scholarly and well-written article on test bias, written by Dr. Norman Frederiksen of the Educational Testing Service.* In it, the author points to another strong advantage of the change-the-test strategy in reformation of curricula. One of the most potent methods to change the way students learn and the way faculty teach is to change the test. Frederiksen's paper reinforces many of the participants' concerns about the use of NBME examinations. The boards are probably a chief reason that the memorization of a large body of facts is a principal educational activity of students. Many faculty offer the NBME examinations as an excuse for lectures presenting a wide range of facts from their particular disciplines. Therefore, relevant changes in education might occur if a national examination were designed to measure the competencies we would like to see in medical students, rather than memorization of detail.

Instead of teaching to the examinations of the NBME, the faculty would have to teach to a performance examination that tested problem-solving, decision-making, self-initiated study, information management, cost awareness and sensitivity to the whole patient. Emphasis would be on assessing application of these competencies in a functional context of patient care. This change in the assessment of medical students would also influence the way in which students learn, as they would realize that

---

* N. Frederiksen, "The Real Test Bias," *American Psychologist* 39(1984):193-202.

the memorization of a large body of facts does not lead to a successful performance on such a certifying examination. They would have to develop the skills and behaviors that are more important to being a physician. The students would also exert pressure on the faculty to provide an educational method more relevant to this kind of certifying examination. The faculty could no longer use the NBME examinations as an excuse for the way they are presently teaching.

This approach also would eliminate the need to design or prescribe specific curricular changes or teaching methods for all medical schools. It would allow each school to meet the challenge of producing the appropriate capabilities in its students in its own way. The skills tested in this certifying examination could make possible a profitable comparison of the effectiveness of different educational approaches in providing the competencies we want to see in graduating students. Replacing the NBME examinations with such a new certifying examination would also encourage schools to use similar, more relevant examinations to evaluate student progress.

The creation of this more relevant certifying examination should ensure that changes in medical education will actually occur and endure. To maintain pride in their schools, the faculty would have to prepare their students in such a way that the students would do well year after year.

I have always been concerned that the commercial airlines might, because of convenience and lower cost, change their assessment procedures. My personal nightmare is that they would move to the assessment methods presently used in most medical schools. Imagine being told that the pilot on your next flight is fresh out of commercial aviation school but that you needn't worry, because he obtained higher than average scores on the examination of the National Board of Aviation Examiners (NBAE), a written objective test with multiple choice, true-false and matching questions. This written test also has some AMPs (Airline Management Problems) in which the pilot manages some of the problems that might occur in flight by choosing the appropriate actions from a list of possible actions. I'm sure you would not be reassured; you would rather know if the pilot can take off, get to your expected destination, land and handle any unexpected problems that might happen in the

course of the flight. Fortunately, the airlines use simulated cock-
pits and real flight assessment methods. We should do no less
for the public who will be the recipients of our graduating students' health care skills.

Therefore, changing the NBME examinations, or substitut-
ing another national certifying examination that does measure
the types of performances we would like to see in graduating
medical students, would not only allow faculty to recognize
problems in medical education, but would also influence the
ways faculty teach and medical students learn.

The Conference Agenda

To reiterate briefly, I am suggesting that:

1. We don't want our efforts and concerns to suffer the same
fate as the efforts of prior dedicated groups over the last fifty
years who have met, worked and published their proceedings
with little effort. We want to formulate and implement strong
moves.
2. We should identify the problems that exist as a result of the
present predominant methods of education, not just list or prescribe putative solutions.
3. Internal strategies brought about by deans or a cadre of educational revolutionaries are probably weak moves, as the many
factors resisting change are difficult to suppress and can defeat
these internal pressures.
4. External agencies that may effect change through funding,
political pressure and accreditation probably represent stronger
and more lasting moves.
5. One of the most effective strategies may be to replace the present NBME examinations with a more relevant examination for
certification of student performance in medical schools, since:
  a. Inappropriate use of the present NBME examinations is
  responsible for many of the present teaching/learning abuses
  involving the memorization of large numbers of facts for
  their own sake.
  b. The deficiencies with present curricular practices would
  become apparent to medical school faculty.
  c. Changing the examination would have a well-established ef-

fect on faculty teaching and student learning, which would lead to the desired reformation.

d. Each school could solve its curricular problems in its own way to produce appropriately skilled and knowledgeable students.

e. Institutional pride would be based on appropriate medical student skills.

f. Medical faculty might be stimulated to use the more relevant testing methods of this examination to evaluate student progress in their curricula.

These assumptions would, in turn, suggest the following agenda:

Thursday, June 14, 1984

Session I: What are the problems that suggest reform of medical education is needed?

Session II: What influences internal to the medical school can be used to encourage curriculum reform, and how can they be put into place?

Session III: What are the external forces that can facilitate educational reform within the medical school?

Friday, June 15, 1984

Session IV: Should a more comprehensive, performance-based certifying examination be developed to replace the present NBME Part I and II examinations? Who should do this? What would be appropriate action steps?

Session I: What Are the Problems That Suggest Reform of Medical Education Is Needed?

The conference was opened with a welcome from Dean Moy of the Southern Illinois University School of Medicine. He explained that the concept for this colloquium originated late in 1982, as those in the medical school began to contemplate the commencement of the institution's tenth graduating class in June of 1984. There was strong feeling that the school should do something significant in concert with this event. Since SIU's "long suit" has been curricular design, a conference on curricular issues seemed appropriate, particularly in light of the considerable recent ferment about problems that exist in medical school curricula. Dean Moy cited the prior Macy Conference on *The New Biology and Medical Education;* the current AAMC project, *Emerging Perspectives on the General Professional Education of the Physician;* and the Institute of Medicine study on *Medical Education and Societal Needs* as significant expressions of concern regarding medical curricula.

Conference participants were exhorted to accept the diagnosis that serious "curriculopathies" exist and to recognize that what is needed now are guidelines by which schools can move towards appropriate changes. Because a mix of theory and practice seemed appropriate in considerations of such reform, Dean Moy explained, participants in this conference were selected to include people who have been active in education and educational reform, as well as senior faculty from traditional schools who must deal with traditional faculty. He pointed out that the task of curricular design was easy for SIU because it started with a new medical school. There were no traditions to be changed. He emphasized that participants in this conference share a common commitment to educational reform. Concluding his remarks,

Dean Moy noted that, because this is the first conference to focus on *where* to start, the participants must operate under Sergeant Preston's Law: The lead dog does most of the work, but he is the only one with a view.

Dr. Hirsch welcomed the participants on behalf of the Macy Foundation. He underlined the foundation's interest in reforming medical education and reminded the group that the present complaints about medical education are identical to those of thirty years ago. Even though there have been significant changes in the practice of medicine over the years, many of the problems in the educational process remain unchanged. Dr. Hirsch noted that many of those who are responsible for existing innovations in medical education are participants in this conference. Reiterating the theme of the meeting, Dr. Hirsch challenged the group to consider not *what* should be done, but *how* it should be done.

Following these introductory remarks, participants were asked to address the topic of this opening session: *What are the Problems That Suggest Reform of Medical Education Is Needed?*

Faculty Complacency

The first issue raised by the group was faculty complacency, also described as a general lack of awareness that there are significant problems in medical education. Because a large number of faculty do not acknowledge that any troublesome areas exist, the problems in the medical education process must be stated persuasively and supported by evidence. The situation is complicated by the fact that the performance or "people skills" that are vitally important in the education of the physician are difficult to test; consequently, inadequacies in medical education are hard to demonstrate.

Absence of Data on Competency of Graduates

The second problem considered by the group was the competency with which physicians now graduating from medical school provide medical care. A principal problem in analyzing physician performance is the lack of objective data; most information on performance is anecdotal. We do not have sufficient data even to make distinctions among graduates from U.S.

schools, American graduates of schools in other countries, and foreign physicians trained outside the U.S. Several participants noted that in the absence of such data, this group could only express opinions about physician performance. It is true that there may be little link between what is observed in a graduate's practice performance and his or her undergraduate educational experience. However, a study conducted at McMaster University demonstrated that the most significant factor in determining the quality of care of hypertensive patients was the year the physician graduated from medical school.* While the AAMC hopes to begin tracking student performance through graduation, the problem of accurately measuring clinical performance after graduation must be resolved if these data are to be meaningful. One member of the group commented that we now have the technology, if not the political power, to document what does happen in practice; simulated patients and patient instructors are capable of providing such documentation. Even though increasingly more and better data on the performance of physicians may be available, it cannot be assumed that undergraduate medical education has a significant influence on performance. Other factors such as residency training, continuing medical education and practice environment may be equally important.

Judging the Adequacy of Current General Medical Education

The discussion then moved to a consideration of the appropriateness or adequacy of current undergraduate medical education. The fact that students spend four years in undergraduate medical education and come out as good physicians does not necessarily mean that those undergraduate years were used appropriately to prepare the students for their future tasks. The very real problems and complexities involved in providing a general medical education should be considered carefully. There is great heterogeneity among physicians in different specialty practices; it is difficult to identify those elements of undergraduate education which are common to all physicians. Since professional education beyond medical school becomes more discrete and

---

* D. L. Sackett, R. B. Haynes, E. S. Gibson, et al., "Randomised Clinical Trial for Improving Medication Compliance in Primary Hypertension," *Lancet* 1 (1975):1205-08.

specialized, the adequacy of the general medical education in the undergraduate years cannot be judged on the basis of later performance. It is also much easier to determine an appropriate education for specialty study than for general undergraduate medical studies. Several participants agreed that the problem of general medical education demands more attention in medical schools.

Preparing Students for Future Practice

The next problem area addressed by the group was the extent to which medical curricula prepare students for future practice. This discussion was prefaced by the observation that, by most existing standards, medicine has been very successful. There is no difficulty in placing graduates, and students still want to come to medical school. However, according to one participant, some fundamental aspects of the educational process can be taken as wrong on face value. Medical students and residents dislike their educational experiences. There is no preparation for self-learning. Most importantly, however, there is no preparation for the challenges and changes that will occur in medical practice in the future. Medical schools have an obligation to look at what the world will need in ten years so that today's students, who will be entering a practice a decade from now, will be appropriately prepared. Many participants stressed that this factor alone is a highly compelling reason for curricular reform, even when good data on physician performance do not exist. Present curricula do not adequately prepare students for the significant changes occurring in medicine. One group member noted that in the future, many more graduates will be members of corporations, working in teams rather than in the current solo practice environment. The for-profit need to cut costs will conflict with the physician's concern for appropriate care of the patient's problem. Because the physician will have too vested an interest, the control of health care quality may become the concern of a third party.

The participants noted several other subjects that must be given attention in undergraduate medical education if contemporary problems in health care are to be addressed: 1) appropriate use of drugs; 2) genetic screening; 3) care of the elderly; 4) nutrition; 5) management of chronic problems; 6) decision-making involving alternative medical therapies; 7) cost-effective health care; 8) health maintenance; 9) preventive care; and 10) interpersonal skills. Regarding this last topic, there was an interesting and perceptive exchange between two participants. One asked, "Can we teach compassion?", to which the other replied, "No, but we can *inhibit* it."

Towards the end of this session one dean indicated that most students and graduates display no apparent problems and seem to do well despite all the concerns expressed. In response, another dean pointed out that medical students are generally so bright that they will do well despite the curriculum. He further noted that such anecdotal assessments can be beguiling, preventing a careful look at the performance of all students and the quality of the curriculum.

Ideas Generated in Summary of Session I

With the support and encouragement of the group, Dr. Moore and Dr. Neufeld summarized the ideas generated in this first session that might be used to argue for reform of the medical curriculum. The two summaries are synthesized as follows:

The purpose of medical education is to prepare physicians for the effective, life-long practice of medicine. Significant changes in the scientific basis for the practice of medicine and in the social, political and environmental trends affecting medical care have led to significant modifications in the educational experience of the physician. Among these were the Flexner Report, federally financed research which enriched the content of medical education, the growth of the hospital and extended residency program as an integral part of education prior to practice, and the rapid subspecialization of medicine with its enhanced needs for biotechnical skills. On what evidence do we base a contemporary conclusion that medical education is, once again, in need of significant reform?

While generally acknowledging that the medical care system of this country is among the best in the world, critics point out disturbing but scattered evidence from medical practice which suggests that the educational process might warrant

modification. Documented misuse of drugs, wide and unex-
plainable inter-physician variation in the use of tests and diagnostic procedures, and the documented consumer dissatisfaction with medical services provide direct evidence supporting
a serious re-examination of the means by which medical education could be changed to improve the performance of practicing physicians. It is difficult to clearly attribute that performance to the undergraduate medical education experience,
however; it is more likely that physician performance is a product of the post-graduate experience and of the practice environment. Nevertheless, careful attention to the general education of the medical student in the undergraduate period may
go some ways towards the correction of these problems. It is
important to prepare a summary of what is known about and
expected in physician performance.

A second line of reasoning that argues we should not accept
certain aspects of current medical education rests on *prima
facie* evidence. Even a superficial examination of the educational process yields the conclusion that the curricula of today's medical schools are overcrowded. There is no systematic
method of culling outdated information and adding new information. There is little attention to helping students learn
the skills of information management. Students are generally
not engaged in active learning which could provide them with
an opportunity to develop skills of life-long independent learning, critical analysis and self-evaluation. Many, if not most,
medical students and residents find their educational experiences grinding and unpleasant. The educational methodolo-
gies utilized are generally not consistent with what we know
about adult learning. Physicians could be better prepared to
withstand the emotional stresses of practice.

Finally, and perhaps most persuasively, we are entering a
period of unprecedented and rapid change in medicine. Developments in the practice of medicine in the next ten to twenty
years will require substantial revisions of medical curricula.
The biologic-scientific basis of medical care is undergoing
fundamental revision leading to radically new conceptions of
how we diagnose and treat disease. Health beliefs and public
attitudes about health and medical care are changing rapidly.
Demographically, as the population ages, the incidence of ag-

ing will increase. Massive change in financing and delivering medical care is occurring. Financially, the primary focus is on reducing health care costs to government and business. Delivery of medical care is increasingly shifting towards a for-profit, business orientation. These changes are already yielding environmental modifications which will create a world of practice quite different from that of today. The for-profit need to cut costs will conflict with the physician's concern for appropriate care of the patient's problem.

Medical education must adapt its methods to produce graduates with the requisite skills, knowledge, concerns for patients and thinking abilities to enable them to perform effectively and efficiently in these changing circumstances. The increased need to attend to illness prevention and health promotion, the need to carefully attend to the scientific and efficient use of new technology, the need to consider how the "caring function" of physicians as patient advocates in the new health care system can be carried out, the ethics that guide the decisions of physicians in the context of new technology and the rapidly-changing health care settings—these environmental factors demand new skills and attitudes not taught conventionally.

For these three reasons—because documented problems in physician performance do exist; because current medical curricula are clearly overloaded with outdated information and do not facilitate the development of skills necessary for lifelong independent learning, critical analysis and self-evaluation; and because dramatic changes now occurring in the medical practice environment will have tremendous impact on patient care in the future—we believe medical education is at a critical juncture and that fundamental reevaluation and revision are necessary.

Session II: What Influences Internal to the Medical School Can Be Used to Encourage Curricular Reform, and How Can They Be Put into Place?

Potential internal influences for curricular change were considered in the second session of the conference. The group quickly moved into a discussion of the possible motivation of deans for curricular reform, first questioning whether deans of medical schools do recognize that a problem exists. Several participants commented that, even when deans do recognize that there is a problem, educational reform often may not be their highest priority. Deans' other priorities include finances, hospital relations, departmental leadership and the future support and development of research programs. Since these problems never disappear completely, there must be some mechanism to constantly call attention to curricular needs. However, one dean noted that his school feels a sense of competition for good applicants, which has caused the institution to be concerned about the attractiveness of its curriculum.

One dean felt that it is strategically easier for deans to respond to external pressures, rather than initiate internal moves for educational reform. When the pressure for educational reform comes from the dean's office, a we—they confrontation between the dean and faculty often occurs. Outside pressure can unite the dean and faculty in a common purpose. Citing the GPEP report as an example, one dean commented that there has been too much criticism of current medical education practices. This criticism suggests that faculty, despite all their efforts, have been doing a very poor job. This dean further suggested that a more positive and acceptable method of generating reform might be to couch the pressure in terms of needs to adapt to future changes in medical practice.

Another potent lever for curricular reform is the residency selection process. The current stress on class rank and NBME examination scores, particularly Part I, tends to reinforce the existing educational abuses in the undergraduate curriculum. If residency directors were compelled to use more relevant criteria such as clinical performance in their selection of residents, schools in turn would be compelled to provide a more relevant assessment of their students. Some residency directors are beginning to explore the possibility of using more relevant assessment methods: one medical school department used simulated patients to evaluate its residency candidates in an attempt to obtain more meaningful information on their abilities.

It was suggested that deans should consider the need for educational reform whenever new chairmen are selected. The extent to which chairmen regard education as an important priority is a vital factor in educational reform.

Rewards for Teaching

Another potential stimulus for change is data on faculty performance, the quality and quantity of teaching. Such information might motivate deans and chairmen to consider educational modifications. Curricular reform can also be encouraged by the establishment of a system to reward the effective teacher, and teaching efforts should be supported in the budget and rewarded in tenure and promotion decisions. The budget crunch that has affected most medical schools has had a particularly detrimental effect on departments or offices of medical education, as many institutions perceive this to be one area that can be sacrificed in order to minimize budgetary damage to other medical school departments.

Even though medical schools seem to be markedly different in many respects, one participant observed that the value systems of faculties are quite homogeneous. Research productivity and publications are rewarded, not teaching. Prizes for teaching, such as the Golden Apple award, do not get a faculty member promoted. Advancement is by peer review, not by the dean's priorities. If these disincentives for teaching are to be overcome, ideally there must be a restructuring of the reward system that will promote and support educational efforts through means similar to those by which research and patient care are support-ed. Talented and creative people whose experience is in the area of education should be put in strong positions within the medi-cal school.

A restructuring could also include programmatic budgeting for medical education. Within the faculty, an organization that is responsible for supervising the overall curriculum should exist. Again, continuous monitoring of student and faculty perfor-mance is needed in curricular reform, and feedback must be given frequently and systematically to those involved. One method of initiating such restructuring might be through a gen-eral faculty review of the curriculum. Such a careful examina-tion would give the faculty an awareness of the entire curricu-lum, something most faculty do not perceive under present cir-cumstances, and could get them involved in the impetus for educational reform.

One participant pointed out that although many of these suggested methods for introducing change have been tried in medical schools over the years, they cannot substitute for the more tangible rewards of research and patient service. The per-sonal rewards for teaching in medical school are also quite dif-ferent from those for teaching in graduate education programs. Non-clinical educators receive satisfaction from teaching gradu-ate students, with whom they have a prolonged contact, and whose professional development they can see. Similarly, clinical faculty find it more rewarding to work with residents. Compar-able satisfaction usually is not derived from teaching undergrad-uate medical students.

One dean stated that there is no marketplace for master teachers; schools do not try to steal them or lure them away from other schools. Faculty who become master teachers at one school are likely to be there forever. This viewpoint was not shared by one participant who commented that at his institution, which enjoys the reputation of being a highly innovative school, master teachers are being hired away by other schools all the time.

The Role of Faculty in General Medical Education

The group then considered how teaching faculty should

perform in medical education. It was noted that, although there are many good teachers on faculties, most of them are more enthusiastic than skilled. Faculty tend to teach from the perspective of their own specialties. There is a tendency for faculty to feel that, since they are experts, they obviously know how to teach in their own areas. Participants agreed that mechanisms are needed to enhance the general medical educational skills of faculty members.

One person suggested that schools should try to decrease the separation of traditional research/graduate faculty from undergraduate faculty by contracts that create a blend; for example, faculty members might be committed contractually to 60% research and 40% general medical education. Within the 40% devoted to medical education, faculty efforts should involve purely educational activities and should not be diluted with residency training or other institutional activities. Another participant offered a further distinction between general medical education activities or skills and activities which require more specialized, expert input from faculty. For example, tutoring may be considered an example of general medical education activity in that the faculty teacher facilitates the learning process and is not expected to be a resource for information. In contrast, the resource faculty person serves as an information resource for specialized expertise in his or her area of research or study. This distinction is exemplified in the McMaster University program. The docent system used by the University of Missouri at Kansas City was cited as another example of a program in which faculty are used in general medical education instead of in their fields of specialization. Harvard, too, is considering the establishment of a series of academic societies representing certain broad educational areas; in these proposed societies, faculty would take on an educational perspective greater than that of their own discipline or speciality.

It was again suggested that medical schools should have a small cadre of leaders in the skills of general medical education. One participant recommended that all faculty become involved in education so that they have more than the usual fleeting contact with the curriculum. Several participants agreed that limited awareness of the curriculum often prevents faculty from realizing that educational problems exist. Many in the group concluded that the faculty's dominant concept of education is dispensing content to the students. Because there are adequate and improving resources for information, the task in general education is not to provide content, but to provide guidance to students; the task is not to *teach,* but to *help students learn.* Faculty should be encouraged to take educational mini-sabbaticals in an effort to improve their skills in this area.

The group also felt there is a strong need for schools to form a more accurate contractual relationship with faculty concerning educational tasks. Often the educational activities expected of faculty are not made clear. A specifically-written contract could provide an incentive for the kind of teaching that is essential to achieve educational reform; furthermore, it would establish pay and tenure incentives because faculty effort would be evaluated against the contractual stipulations.

Restructuring Internal Systems for Change

Despite all these recommendations, many participants felt that internal mechanisms in and of themselves probably are not sufficient to accomplish satisfactory and lasting shifts in faculty teaching skills or perceptions of their responsibilities. However, one participant suggested that internal structures could be more powerful if they were appropriately orchestrated. The existing structures and values within the traditional medical school are powerful and tend to inhibit, rather than promote, change. Any one isolated thrust to effect a change in conventional thinking or habits is usually of short duration, since the existing internal structures tend to bring a system back into the previous configuration. If change is to be successful and lasting, a school must simultaneously align a variety of internal factors in the same direction. A useful model for identifying the various forces that can be manipulated for change is the 7-S framework provided by Peters and Waterman in their recent bestseller, *In Search of Excellence:* 1) Structure; 2) Systems; 3) Style; 4) Staff; 5) Skills; 6) Strategy; 7) Shared Values.*

One member of the group observed that if schools only

---

* T.J. Peters and R.H. Waterman, Jr., *In Search of Excellence* (New York: Harper & Row, 1982).

tinker with changes, they will always be disappointed. Reformation requires a restructuring of all of the systems involved at the same time. It is necessary to break apart the traditional systems so that they—it is hoped—will fall back into the desired new configuration. For example, the lasting and significant curriculum changes that were brought about at what was then Western Reserve University (now Case Western Reserve University) in the 1950s were possible because many factors were restructured simultaneously. There was an opportunity to hire a new faculty, a change in management occurred, and there was a restructuring of the educational process. External financing also supported this change, again demonstrating that external factors are instrumental in orchestrating forces for change.

From this point, the group considered the actual structure of the curriculum and the organization of curricular content. Several participants raised questions concerning the appropriate conceptual basis on which to construct new learning approaches. Should the new curriculum be organized around organ systems? On concepts such as host—defenses? By sets of skills? Any such organization would require a trans-disciplinary restructuring of the faculty and a corporate faculty responsibility for the entire educational program. One participant identified this concern for curricular organization as a principal reason why the problem-solving method has not been accepted; faculty want an overarching conceptual organization of content to unify various parts of the curriculum. Curricula might reasonably be organized around learning outcomes such as problem-solving abilities, life-long learning skills, doctor-patient relationships or interpersonal skills, recognition of the need to learn and technical skills.

A physical facility which supports such a restructuring of the curriculum is also critically important, according to several group members. Facilities such as the Center for Professional Development at Southern Illinois University and the case discussion rooms at the Harvard Business School are striking examples of physical space that supports a methodological approach.

The session concluded with a discussion of the contrast between the traditional department structures in medical school and the kinds of realignments that seem necessary to carry out appropriate educational reform. Participants felt that departments should be maintained as they are because they are the basis of residency and graduate programs. Departmental structure should also be maintained for research purposes. However, it is clear that other structures are needed to achieve medical education reform. The matrix management system at McMaster University was cited as one such method by which departmental integrity can be maintained while the institution is developing a corporate structure to support the educational program.

Session III: What Are the External Forces That Can Facilitate Educational Reform within the Medical School?

The third session of the conference centered on external factors that can work towards reform of medical curricula. To begin, the group listed a variety of such forces: accreditation bodies; the National Board of Medical Examiners (NBME); state licensure societies; external funding agencies; federal initiatives and regulations; specialty societies; university presidents, chancellors and governing boards; public perception of physicians; medical schools and medical centers; and the increasing student awareness of the new demands of the market place.

University Presidents

From this list, the group focused its discussion on several specific forces. The first to be considered was university presidents, who might be encouraged to comment on the need for educational reform, as did President Bok of Harvard. Presidents could challenge medical faculty to develop the same creativity in teaching and learning that they have applied to research and patient services in the past. A colloquium for university presidents might be a valuable and effective stimulus for reform.

The National Board of Medical Examiners

A second potential source of influence considered by the group was the NBME. One participant expressed concern that the board exams are too frequently used as a whipping boy in discussions about educational change. It is the medical school faculty who choose to require these examinations for their students, and it is the same faculty who make up the questions.

One participant commented that it is as if a faculty member goes to an NBME subject committee meeting loaded with questions of wide-ranging minutia and then returns to his or her school and says to students, in effect, "I'm sorry, gang, but I have to teach this stuff; it's required on the boards." This misuse of the board examinations might be inhibited if the NBME refused to provide individual subject scores, reporting only a pass or fail for each student. According to one recent report, 78% of all U.S. medical schools require their students to take either Part I, Part II or both NBME examinations. If a pass/fail system were used, it would be important for the NBME to provide detailed subject scores for those students who failed. Another participant suggested that the NBME could be encouraged to develop examinations that would measure more relevant skills. That agency has already admitted that of the 50 skills it has identified as important in clinical competence, only 12 are measured by its examinations. However, many in the group seemed to feel that it would be extremely difficult to change the NBME examinations, since they seem to be tightly controlled by faculty from the various basic science disciplines.

External and Internal Funding

External funding was the third factor considered by the group, although the discussion immediately moved from external to internal sources. The deans in the group generally agreed that educational funds within medical schools have been subsidizing research, clinical care and residency education. It was suggested that more careful cost accounting of educational cost and effort is necessary. Funds which could facilitate educational reform probably exist already, but they are being used to support other activities. One school, even allowing for a preparation time of eight hours for one hour of contact time, determined that the entire first two years of its medical school could be taught to classes of well over a hundred students each with fewer than ten full-time faculty. Schools may be paying faculty in great excess of the educational activities needed or provided. Another participant described a study in which it was shown that the average faculty contact time with students was only 1.2 hours per week. It was suggested that this contact time could be doubled or tripled without additional teaching dollars; the only cost might be increased faculty discomfort. However, it is misleading to examine only one type of academic activity such as education. While it looks as if a great trimming of funds could occur, the reality is that a large number of faculty are needed to mount diverse research and patient service programs. This complex effort requires a wide collection of talents and expertise, far more than would be necessary for any one activity. Another dean noted that the large proportion of tenured faculty in medical schools also inhibits reallocation of funds.

The group identified two types of costs involved in achieving educational reform: the initial costs for materials and facilities to put the new program in place, and the long-term ongoing costs associated with maintaining the new curriculum. The discussion seemed to indicate that initial costs might be subsidized by external funding sources. As far as the second cost is concerned, there might be no need for new money at all. More teaching time could be required from the present faculty. Several participants agreed that there is a strong need for more accurate cost accounting, which could reveal great disparities between the proportion of dollars given to various departments and their percentage of effort to the educational program. Careful cost accounting is also important if an institution is to verify that any curricular reform undertaken does not, in the long run, cost more than the present programs. One participant seemed to sum up these concerns in his concluding statement, "Tuition and state funds should not be considered as unemployment compensation for faculty between grants."

The Liaison Committee on Medical Education

The last external force to be considered by the group was the Liaison Committee on Medical Education (LCME). The LCME uses the NBME examination scores as a measure of a school's ability to educate medical students because no other comparable national standard is available. The recent LCME draft, *Functions and Structure of a Medical School, Standards for Accreditation of Medical Education Programs Leading to the M.D. Degree,* was discussed. This document makes it clear that the LCME hopes to encourage curricular reform; if adopted, such a document could be an important influence on medical schools. The potential role of the LCME in facilitating educational reform is discussed at length in the summary of Session IV.

Session IV: Can We Develop an Approach to the Evaluation of Medical Student Performance That Might Lead to Appropriate Curricular Reformation?

The final session began with a brief presentation by the moderator. He emphasized that the previous discussions had been focused on a number of important factors that might facilitate change from within the medical school: response to the certain need to prepare students for the type of practice that they will be entering ten to twenty years from now; the development of a systematic approach to educational reformation that realigns budgets, faculty responsibilities and faculty rewards. However, because good NBME examination scores remain a principal source of faculty satisfaction with the status quo, the heavy use of these examinations inhibits motivation for educational reform. With good NBME examination scores, faculty feel there is no problem. NBME scores are frequently used as a criterion for the selection of residents, and furthermore, board scores are the criteria by which external bodies such as the LCME judge the school's curriculum.

Although in previous sessions the group developed new insights regarding reform and suggested new approaches, the moderator noted that many of these are similar to those expressed by previous groups. There is a genuine risk that the deliberations of this group may result solely in a bound volume of proceedings on the shelf, as have the works of previous groups over the past thirty years. In most cases, those conferences in which intelligent and influential minds have convened to express the same concerns have had little effect. The moderator observed that, in their protagonist papers, nearly all of the participants identified problems with the NBME examinations as they are presently used by medical schools. The discussions in this conference have reinforced that perception. Not only are the NBME examination scores seen to be a measure of the school's worth both internally and externally, but the majority of faculty teach to the NBME examinations, and students study in a manner which will enable them to pass, since examination scores are used as criteria for assessing student progress. Most agree that this is not a problem of the National Board of Medical Examiners *per se,* but a problem created by the schools' use of the examinations.

Nevertheless, the NBME examinations do not measure what we wish to see in the physician-to-be, nor do they measure the true value of a school's educational program. There must be tools to measure such abilities as problem-solving, patient care, interpersonal skills, ethical and moral decision-making, emergency care, efficiency and cost-effectiveness. These skills cannot be estimated adequately by a multiple-choice test which requires the student to choose among given options. They should be measured by test performance in a variety of formats which simulate actual experience. The moderator again referred to Frederiksen's article on test bias, in which that author clearly demonstrates how changing the examination can change teaching and learning methods. In the medical arena, the work of Dr. David Newble at the University of Adelaide in Australia demonstrates Frederiksen's thesis.* Dr. Newble was able to change the teaching in the clinical years of medical school by changing the final examination given to students. Such powerful moves are needed to initiate curricular reform. More relevant examinations should reduce complacency and cause faculty to teach essential skills. To succeed in these types of examinations, students must learn in a way that is appropriate for the acquisition of these skills.

One participant agreed that a new force is needed within the medical school to balance the effect of the NBME examinations, the only existing curricular standard by which schools can be compared. Another group member suggested that the LCME could provide vital impetus if, for accreditation, it re-

---

* D.I. Newble and K. Jaeger, "The Effect of Assessments and Examinations on the Learning of Medical Students." *Medical Education* 17(1983):165-171.

quired schools to use a battery of testing methods that assess clinical skills and other competencies valued by faculty.

Many of the testing instruments that assess clinical skills and problem-solving abilities involve simulated patients or cases. According to one member of the group, many faculty are concerned that simulations cannot be used in a national certifying examination because they cannot be used conveniently to assess thousands of students at one time. For this reason the NBME has continued to rely on paper examinations, although it is now considering examinations at multiple computer terminals. Another participant commented that participants were considering testing as if it should occur nationally on one day. More complex testing procedures based on simulations could be used if testing involved smaller groups of students on different days throughout the year. Schools might also be encouraged to develop and use such relevant testing procedures for their own graduates. If so, it was suggested that in this case the schools would have to be supervised in this process. Given this concern about quality control in such testing procedures, one group member suggested that a network of regional centers might be established near clusters of medical schools to develop these elaborate procedures for testing clinical competence.

Another participant pointed out that we criticize the clinical capabilities of foreign graduates when indeed we have no measure of our own students' clinical performance. An alternative suggestion was to encourage the NBME to change its examination process to include some of these more relevant tests of clinical competence. One group member commented that this might be an opportune time to work with the NBME because the Federation Licensing Examination (FLEX) seems to be replacing the licensing function of the NBME. Another participant pointed out that in the past there was a division of interest between the state licensing boards and the medical schools where evaluation was concerned. Because faculties have increasingly adopted the use of licensure-type examinations in the last decade, the faculty role in determining the curriculum has been diminished; the licensure system is driving the educational system and the faculty.

Again it was recommended that the NBME should move to reporting on a straight pass-fail basis so that faculty would be less interested in using the NBME examinations for internal assessment purposes and comparison with other schools. Another group member suggested that a two-step process might be carried out: the NBME could first move to a pass-fail system of reporting and then as a second step begin to change the format of its examinations to utilize instruments that more accurately assess the important components of clinical competence. A panel might be brought together to look at how these instruments might be incorporated into new board examinations.

At this point the group began a lengthy discussion of the feasibility and/or desirability of developing a national standardized examination that would assess the broader range of clinical competencies. Several participants were concerned that less radical changes posed in the past have been defeated on the basis of feasibility alone. It was pointed out that the NBME did start in this direction after the report of its Committee on Goals and Priorities (the *GAP* report)* in June of 1973. The NBME should be encouraged to get back on the track; the technology for these kinds of examinations now exists. There have been significant advances in the methods for evaluating performance, and it is now possible to test for a variety of important skills within clinical competence. Admittedly, this probably would not be possible on any given day in a hundred testing centers across the nation.

One participant reiterated that there is a need to put such evaluation methods in place in medical schools and then feed the results into a national reporting system. These examinations could be scored and reported from a central location. Another member of the group again suggested a network of testing sites, as these evaluation systems may be too elaborate and expensive for each school to develop on its own.

Again the group raised the concern that it may be difficult for the NBME to change. Because most medical schools that have gone to the trouble of developing commencement objectives (specifications of those behaviors and abilities expected of medical students just prior to graduation) have produced rather similar objectives, there may be a sufficient commitment from a

---

* *Evaluation in the Continuum of Medical Education* (Philadelphia: National Board of Medical Examiners, 1973).

variety of medical schools to set up an objectives-based examination in place of the NBME examinations. Over 18,000 medical students graduate each year. If these graduates paid a small testing fee, enough money would be generated to seriously interest a testing agency in developing such an examination. Several group members agreed that agencies other than the NBME might be very creative in this area. Even the NBME might be interested in writing a proposal for developing such an examination. In response to this suggestion, one participant commented that the NBME has the resources to do this, and that, as a leader in evaluation research, it should be asked to assist the schools in developing more relevant evaluation procedures of their own. Because of many vested interests, the politics surrounding the NBME are very difficult. Others in the group felt that the NBME will test anything that can be machine scored, is least expensive and easiest to administer. It was felt that the board is now as open as it ever has been to considering other testing methods. One participant suggested that this group point out that it has no confidence in the present NBME examinations, as they are unidimensional in character while the competencies of concern in medical students are multidimensional. It would be inappropriate to talk about possible alternatives to the present board examination format. As it is now, the certification process is based only on paper and pencil examinations, which are inappropriate. There can be no confidence in what a student *says* he or she will do in a given situation. It is far more important to see that students are capable of actually performing relevant tasks. Any certifying examination for medical students should reflect the reality of the tasks the physician will face in the future.

Reflecting on the problems that followed the GAP report, one dean felt it would be important to question whether polarization can be risked at this time and whether a sufficient number of deans and medical schools would support this type of reform. Although the NBME staff has already indicated willingness to change, it is necessary to obtain the support of the many medical schools before reform can be accomplished. Others in the group were skeptical that there would be sufficient consensus to provide a market for such a new test. The group generally believed that it would be more difficult to get faculty to accept the test than it would be to actually develop the test. To this, one participant proposed compromise involving incremental changes. Initially a complementary assessment to the NBME exams, modest in scope but intended for further development, could be developed. This strategy of incremental add-ons to the board examinations would allow time to continue the development of new assessment methods and to overcome the inertia of tradition.

A group member reemphasized that the NBME, by its own admission, measures only one quarter of what it admits are the critical characteristics of competence; measuring the remaining three quarters of those abilities must be the responsibility of the faculty of the various medical schools. It must be made clear to medical school faculty that their goal is not to make Ph.D.s or board-certified specialists out of their graduates. There are competencies that are far more important to the preparation of a physician than the recall or recognition of extensive minutia in many different subject areas.

One participant noted that the state licensure agencies are now looking for some way to measure the three-quarters of competency not measured by the NBME examinations. State agencies need such tools to evaluate the competency of foreign medical school graduates before they can be permitted to practice medicine. If such examinations were required of foreign graduates, it would only be a short time before legal pressures would require that these examinations be administered to U.S. graduates as well. What is needed is a legal, valid barrier that would allow into the country only those graduates whose capabilities match the skills of U.S. graduates. The need for an instrument that will screen out unacceptable graduates provides a very real political opportunity for the testing instruments discussed here. Another participant commented that it also would be valuable to have such examinations at the end of residency programs.

In light of the above discussion, another group member suggested that the focus should not be on the exam, but on the criteria for accreditation by the LCME. Each school should be required to document that it has commencement objectives for its students and to document how its students are being evaluated. This requirement could provide a legal basis for the evaluation of students educated outside the U.S. From this there might emerge a national instrument which otherwise would be nearly impossible to implement at this time.

Another participant indicated that faculty in many medical schools are uneasy with the present methods of assessing clinical performance. One hundred thirteen schools expressed interest in being involved in the AAMC project concerning needs assessment in the evaluation of clerks; unfortunately, the AAMC currently can work with only eight institutions. As there is little evidence that any reliable assessment system for clinical performance now exists in many medical schools, it might be valuable to concentrate on this faculty uneasiness.

One member of the group then recommended that the LCME formally state that a medical school which requires the Part I NBME examination must justify this use and explain how the scores are used. Furthermore, the LCME might encourage schools to show evidence of assessment procedures that both assure the quality of their graduates and evaluate the curriculum. An even more radical suggestion was that the schools create a separate budget for such evaluation mechanisms to assure the quality of their graduates. Each school might be required to use five percent of its tuition income to develop competency-based assessments which would be conducted by faculty other than those responsible for the curriculum. One participant offered the cautionary note that a uniform national examination may not be advisable, even if it were more relevant, as it could stifle innovation in the various schools. Instead he encouraged the creation of generic mechanisms to enable schools to evaluate the competency of their medical students on their own.

Another participant pointed out that this approach addresses only one of the problems associated with the use of the NBME examinations. Since the NBME examinations are still used as an instrument to evaluate the curriculum of schools as part of the accreditation process, these proposals would not affect that problem. One member suggested that the group urge the NBME to develop procedures to assess competencies beyond the recognition of facts, and that the group urge schools to develop their own exams by broadening the LCME statement. This was followed by a suggestion that licensure examinations and examinations after residency training be performance- or competency-based. Again citing the residency program that used simulated patients to evaluate the abilities of applicants, one parti-pant commented that if all residency program directors required similar kinds of evaluations, this would also have a profound effect on the medical schools. If such competency-based evaluations were used, faculty behavior in the undergraduate curriculum would change and the various post-graduate programs could select better residents. The Educational Commission for Foreign Medical Graduates (ECFMG) is also trying to develop a more performance-oriented examination for foreign medical graduates. This would be followed by the challenge that U.S. graduates would also be required to pass this examination. There was strong feeling that the response of this group should be to encourage local development of such examinations.

The discussion again returned to the NBME and the importance of urging it to report only pass-fail, without separate discipline scores. As a backup, students who fail could be provided with more detailed information regarding the nature of their deficiencies. Furthermore, it was pointed out that if the NBME is not obligated to report individual sub-scores, the examination itself could be made considerably shorter without sacrificing its reliability, thereby making it practical to add other performance measures to the exam.

One educator in the group was again stimulated to point out that the NBME's certifying examination is currently driving the teaching activities of our faculties and the learning activities of our students. He pointed out that the NBME examination in its current format is not an adequate indication of competence, as there is no evidence of the validity of this examination in its relationship to practice. To measure the clinical performance skills of medical graduates, it is necessary to develop a variety of simulation formats. This participant described the military's reliance on simulations during the 1974 fuel shortage. Because of economic considerations, training on simulators was substituted for actual flying time, underlying the value of simulations in teaching and evaluation. The group member then posed a rhetorical question: "Are we confident enough in the NBME examination, in its current format, to consider it in selecting our own private physicians?"

Another educator advised that there should be an open checkbook to build prototype simulations for the evaluation of competency in medicine, although such models might be too costly for a national certification examination. To this reservation, one dean responded by pointing out that in comparison to the cost of educating each medical student (approximately $200,000), and his or her subsequent responsibilities, nothing is too expensive to ensure the quality of graduates.

As the conference moved towards closure, one participant pointed out that this colloquium had begun by stating the problem with medical education and that the discussion was ending with the idea that it was important for schools to set goals for their graduates. While the group had considered ways schools could organize for reformation through the restructuring of budgets and educational responsibility, the participants were now talking about where it is best to enter the objectives—teaching methods—evaluation loop in the educational process. He called for another conference to demonstrate practical evaluation formats that faculty could take back to their institutions to improve their assessment of student competence. He also suggested that the group encourage the LCME to require medical schools to set up evaluation methods against their common objectives. The same group member also suggested a different conference for the purpose of generating new ideas about evaluation and disseminating already-tested or established methods. In response to this, another participant proposed that such an evaluation conference could be held on a regional basis and should involve teaching faculty. Another person in the group added that schools using NBME examinations should be told that it is inappropriate to use these exams for internal assessment when students are required to pass. Another added that all examinations used by schools should assess the ability to apply information, not just the ability to recognize it.

At this point one participant said that he was now convinced that there are practical ways to expand the measurement of competency. He further recommended that medical schools should be developing these types of assessments and that faculty take the responsibility for this development within the various schools. He also encouraged the group to move quickly in this regard and stated that his organization would support the effort.

Another member of the group pointed out that the new pressures to be faced by graduates in the next decades, pressures of financial and cost-containment strategies, raise the need to add moral and ethical components to the commencement objectives. These will be essential skills in the physician of the future. If for-profit arrangements become more prevalent, physicians' responsibility for the indigent and the poor also will become an increasing concern. He further suggested that students should perhaps go into a general medical service on graduation, caring for the indigent and the poor before going into specialty training. This interim experience would unlock the tracking into specialties that occurs at the present time. As evidence of the pragmatic aspects of this approach to specialty training, the participant pointed out that most business schools require students to work three or four years in the field before beginning graduate studies.

One member of the group commented that he thought the group had not dealt in sufficient detail with the specific changes that must be undertaken within medical schools to cause a change in the curriculum, to overcome the impediments for change and to maintain the change. He recommended that another conference be held to deal with these strategies in greater depth and to consider how they are to be undertaken with no increase in funds. Mechanisms for faculty reward and recognition for educational activities should also be considered in this proposed conference.

Dr. Hirsch closed the meeting, reminding the group that they had been invited for two reasons: 1) to consider ways to reform the curriculum; and 2) to celebrate the commencement of SIU's tenth graduating class. He pointed out that it may be easier to start reforms in new schools, citing McMaster and Southern Illinois University as two examples of new approaches to medical education. While their final stories are not in, they seem to be highly successful to date. They demonstrate the kinds of things that many would like to see happen in other schools. For older schools, curriculum reform is not easy. Perhaps the best approach is to encourage the faculty to review what they are doing, in spite of their perceptions of success. Dr. Hirsch noted that Harvard is the best example of a school that is reexamining what it is doing. That reexamination has led to a wide publicizing of medical curriculum reformation issues, which may encourage other traditional schools to do the same. He concluded with an observation that he had found this meeting interesting and stimulating, but had not expected that specific answers would come out of it. However, he said, if all the conference accomplishes is to convince other schools to take a fresh look at medical education, the meeting will have been highly successful.

Appendix A:
Protagonist Papers

The Reformation Movement in Medical Education
Must There Be Martyrs?

Stephen Abrahamson, Ph.D.

During the three decades from the Flexner Report to the turmoil of World War II, American medical education's faith in its educational philosophy and practices grew ever stronger. Because of the experiences of medical schools during those war years in the use of accelerated programs, voices of apostates were heard in the land, asking whether there might indeed be other approaches—of shorter duration, less demanding rote memory, with more emphasis on continuity of care. With the end of the war and the beginning of the remarkable era of medical school subsidy by the National Institutes of Health, medical education entered its own "renaissance," with increasingly ardent allegiance to basic Flexnerian principles—unfortunately without critical re-examination of those princples and the way in which they were being interpreted by those invoking them in curriculum-development discussions. Indeed, the very mention of Flexner could serve to stifle honest questioning of educational practices; and shibboleths rather than inquiry guided curriculum planning.

At long last, albeit for perhaps the wrong reasons, a significant movement is now being sensed: it is time to "reform" medical education. But such a movement will meet with stern resistance, if history and politics can serve as reminders. While reformation of American medical education might not beget the literal bloodshed of the Protestant Reformation, it undoubtedly will precipitate some of the most agonizing moments in higher education as institutionally entrenched—almost sacred—practices are challenged, and thus—in the eyes of many—threatened. Debates, far from being academic and intellectual, will be all-too-often emotional and one can anticipate figurative bloodshed in the form of destruction of promising academic careers of those who are perceived by established medical education as "threatening" when, in fact, they are "challenging" by merely raising questions. But it does seem clear: from the development of this medical education "religion" through its own "renaissance," it is now entering its "reformation."

Can anything be gleaned from history, from political science, from management science, to help avoid the trauma associated with a reform movement? Or are we doomed to repeat history and produce a new set of martyrs whose major sin is to question the educational *status quo*? Unfortunately, medical education already has many illustrations of martyrdom—or near-martyrdom—of those who "dared" to raise question. What has been the fate of the person who first challenged the viability of a memory-based practice of medicine in this era of the "knowledge explosion?" Far from being nominated for the Flexner Award of the AAMC, far from being idolized as a leader in American medical education, this person is slowly being academically extinguished for his pains. And in another example, what was the medical education establishment's response to the recommendations of the "GAP Committee" of the National Board of Medical Examiners? Instead of the expected intellectual and academic discussion, there was much behind-the-scene politicking and podium posturing all designed to preserve unthinking obeisance to medical education shibboleths.

If medical education is truly at the point of considering "reform," a movement obviously involving "change," much can be gained by careful consideration of the phenomenon of social change—that is, the *process* of change, as opposed to preoccupation with the *content* of that change. American medical education, like any other institution in our society, has an organizational life. And, like any other organization, it manifests built-in energies working for its own perpetuation: a natural resistance to change; vested interests of those whose lives might not be so rewarding if change occurs; and a self-serving power structure to guard against change. Indeed, one must consider a number of factors opposing change: human factors and institutional factors.

Human Factors Opposing Change. The first of these is *complacency*, a feeling of secure—almost smug—self-satisfaction. American medical education almost justifiably has this characteristic—but, unfortunately, to excess. On the one hand, there is reason for some self-satisfaction: years of acceptable performance of an increasing number of medical schools with greatly increased enrollments, production of the nation's physicians at levels of competence more than equal to the tasks they perform. But complacency is defined by Webster as ". . . self-satisfaction accompanied by unawareness of actual dangers or deficiencies." Those who sense possible "dangers or deficiencies" and raise questions are treated to murmurs of complacency as a form of defense—indeed, the first line of a rather intricate defense.

The next human factor to be considered is that of *habit*. More often than not, when one questions a medical education practice, the response is one of surprise: "How can you question something that we have always done?" In fact, too much of medical education teaching practices seem to be a matter of ritual. Behaviors that are automatic and long-unquestioned are difficult enough to change. When those same habits are part of the total educational scheme, the difficulty is greatly magnified.

Still one more factor is probably best described by the phrase, *"But it worked for us before."* Somewhat related to complacency, the difference is that here the resistance is based on almost personal testimony: "After all, I went through it and I turned out all right." In other words, because the present system has been successful in the past, one must not question it; one must not even wonder whether there might be a "better way."

Selective perception is still one more human factor opposing change. All too often, we tend to see things (hear things) which support our own points of view. Thus we "see" the thousands of currently practicing physicians; we read of the improvements in health-care practices; we hear of the high level of health of the American citizen. But we tend *not* to see the number of impaired physicians and not to acknowledge the less-than-optimum care provided by some physicians; we *forget* the many instances of physicians who are not cognizant of or applying the improvements in practice; we *don't* want to hear of the significant number of health-care-disenfranchised Americans. Therefore, with selective perception supporting them, many defend practices of medical education by selectively rejecting evidence of less-than-good results.

Finally, as is the case in any human endeavor, there is the factor of *ego involvement.* It is, after all, human beings who are doing the teaching, the testing, the curriculum planning. Any question of program adequacy immediately attacks those who are involved. All too often one discovers that the person who has been lecturing on a given topic also has come to believe it is important—even when his first involvement in that little teaching exercise might have been reluctant or even when his first involvement might have been perceived by himself as not very important in the greater scheme of things.

But these are only "human" factors. Institutions have a life of their own—undoubtedly related to the individuals who are part of them. And a quick examination of some of those factors will reveal the relationship between "human" and "institutional" factors.

Institutional Factors Opposing Change. The first of these factors is *xenophobia,* the fear of anything alien or strange. Suggestions for resistance which increases geometrically in relation to the strangeness of the new ideas. If the change is purely cosmetic, the institution reacts with only a little resistance—and that much probably from certain individuals. Even if that modification, however, involves only the shifting of large blocks of time from one year to another, then the institutional reaction is more than just wariness—and it is widespread, not coming just from individuals. But when the suggestion involves a radical new look, individuals and departments close ranks. Indeed, during the sixties and seventies, when many special schools were attempting to modify their curricula to better meet perceived needs of society and students, changes often began as radical, quite different, innovations but ended up as cosmetic repairs perhaps involving some shift in the building blocks.

The institution frankly resists any perceived *threat to comfortable patterns*—the second of the institutional factors. There are institutional behaviors involving decision-making, educational planning, program evaluation, student assessment, registration, class scheduling, and the like. Imagine the *institutional* reaction to a plan that involves no lectures and no formally scheduled courses! Quite aside from the reaction of *individuals* within the school, there would be a *collective* resistance because of the disturbance of set patterns. Institutionalization has been described and discussed in the literature of sociology but it has not been reckoned with very well in medical education.

Along with the threat to institutional patterns of behavior, there is the factor of *institutional structure*. It is no secret that one of the major resistances of American medical schools to even consider the worth of the then-novel Western Reserve plan of the early 1950's was the rigidity of departmental structure. Indeed, many of Abrahamson's "Diseases of the Curriculum" are caused and/or agravated by the departmental structure existing in almost all American medical schools. Any number of medical schools truly failed in their attempt to change to an organ-system approach to the teaching of basic sciences because of their inability to provide a structure that would facilitate communication among the several departments.

A natural follow-on is the factor of *vested interests* which are threatened by suggestions of change. Worse than it might have been had the pre-war conditions simply continued—with all of the same building of vested interests—consider the situation after three decades of ever-increasing financial support of schools and departments by the extramural program of the NIH. It is not unusual to find schools which are totally dependent upon such funds; and departments have been known to exist by being supported well in excess of fifty percent by "soft money," that is, outside funding sources. Now, with some contraction of availability of funds, departments are feeling threatened and naturally fall back on their claim of importance to the educational efforts of the institution. Suggestion for change threatens those pockets of vested interest. Part of the reaction against the concept of a single examination for licensure (to be administered at the interface between undergraduate education and house-officer service) was blatantly stated by associations of professors of various basic sciences: any such move will depreciate the *status* of basic science departments in medical schools.

Another factor is that of the *domino theory* being applied to medical schools. The thinking is simple: watch out, "they" begin by making a little change here or there, and the next thing you know, "they" want to change everything. Indeed, there are many instances of resistance to change which clearly grow out of this domino theory. Discussions at the executive committee level (i.e., department heads) frequently show a closing of the ranks when one or another department is threatened. Where discussion begins to focus on the probability of institutional advantage to the elimination of a given academic department, other units feel the threat (they may be "next") and unite in support of that department, clearly providing evidence of the truth of the maxim: "If the Edsel Division of the Ford Motor Company had been a department in an American medical school, it would still be there."

The final factor opposing change in a medical school is that of *guilt by association*. Many institutional efforts have foundered when one (or more) of the persons interested in change acquires the reputation of being "radical" or "idealistic." Once such a phenomenon occurs, then any other person who becomes interested in the *ideas* (not the radical person) is perceived as being "one of that kind." The institution, again through its structure and patterns of activities, places pressure on would-be reformers by condemning them as guilty by association with that radical or that idealist. This kind of institutional reaction is, of course, a classic manifestation of resistance to change—one without rationality, nutured by emotional response . . . but this time as an institution, not by individuals.

Considering the theme of this essay, one might at this point offer a response to the original question, "do there have to be martyrs?" That answer would, of course, be "yes" since the collection of human and institutional factors opposing change is so forbidding. The logic in support of those factors is equally impressive, coming from the sciences of management, politics, and administration. The question is whether any steps might be taken to ensure a more favorable response to invitations to consider change. And there are some logical preventive measures to be reviewed.

Facilitation of Innovation. The suggestions listed below are not arranged in any special order (e.g., importance, logical sequence) but are offered for consideration.

1. *Know the system.* Change ought never to be proposed unless those who are proponents are thoroughly familiar with the institution and its patterns of behaving and its structure. Knowing how the institution is governed is essential: Who makes the

decisions? Who are required to approve change? What is the committee structure? How are schedules prepared? Who scores examinations? It is important to know both the formal-covert-structure and behavior patterns *and* the informal-covert-structure and patterns of behavior. Where is the "real" power in the school? How strong is each department? What is the nature of the communication grapevine?

2. *Anticipate problems and resistance.* If one knows which people will be the most troublesome—and why—there is a much better chance of planning to account for that resistance. Those who are promoting consideration of change would do well to meet and literally list the potential sources of trouble along with the specific line of resistance anticipated. It would be even better to add the reasons for that expected resistance. Some might consider this kind of preventive measure to be potentially inflammatory or even the beginning of a self-fulfilling prophesy. To the contrary, it is the realistic side of the idealism of reform. How foolish it is to find a mean pocket of resistance and then say, "I just knew these guys would react this way!" How wise it would have been to anticipate (correctly, it is to be hoped!) the problems and to plan for their management beforehand.

3. *Modify the organization for the innovation.* One of the most important lessons to be learned from the Western Reserve curriculum change thirty-odd years ago is that the organization was significantly changed in order to accommodate the new educational planning demands placed on the faculty by the shift to organ-system orientation for the teaching of basic sciences. Many schools attempting to follow the form of that curriculum innovation found themselves unable to realize the full potential of that approach because no changes were made in the organization: its structure and patterns of function. Then, when a "teaching committee" made its plans, department heads would balk at implementation (for which they felt responsible), and the program would find itself in deep trouble. Similarly, decisions about *when* certain teaching was to take place and *who* was to do the teaching would become a bone of contention, with the teaching committee and the department head each claiming that the power was vested in them. As another example, how much more difficult would it be (if not impossible) for a school with a strong departmental structure to attempt a totally integrated, problem-based

curriculum! David Maddison certainly anticipated that problem in Newcastle and took steps to minimize the negative effects of departmentalization.

4. *Obtain administrative support.* Despite the accurate claim that many department heads have more power (money) at their own discretion than the dean does, administrative support is essential for curriculum change to take place. Not only must there be the academic and moral support from the chief administrative officer of the school, there must also be the necessary resources supplied by the administration. Whatever form the change takes, new materials will be needed ($), planning time will be needed ($), faculty orientation will be needed ($), student recruitment will be needed ($). Full, enthusiastic administrative support is essential— probably including administrative figures other than the dean . . . both above and below in the institutional organization.

5. *All parties must be (or at least feel) involved.* As planning begins, care must be taken to involve everyone: administrators, students, and particularly the faculty. Not only must the committee members, themselves, be active participants, others must also be invited to contribute ideas and reactions. Obviously, most medical school faculties are of such a size that some form of representation must be utilized to facilitate the curriculum-planning processes. But care must be taken to have all faculty members feel that they have been involved and/or consulted. Of course, even the best efforts may fail. In one school, for instance, two department chairmen refused to assist in the implementation of a new curriculum, stating that they had never been consulted, when in fact one of them had served on the very curriculum committee that had planned the change and the other had been chairman of that same committee! Both had been active members and had had a significant influence on the outcome of the five-year planning effort. However, some of their ideas had *not* been incorporated into the final design which—in turn —had been approved by total consensus of the committee (actually a unanimous vote . . . including those two) before being acted on further. While this is an extreme example, it is not that farfetched. Involvement of everybody is essential at all stages. In another school, for example, one committee member (a departmental head, again) refused to have members of his department discuss the planning until it was "further along." By that time,

the committee was pleased with their processes and results and found themselves defending ideas against the bitter attacks of members of that department who felt that all these things had been done "behind their backs."

6. *Changes must be consistent with the value system.* On the surface, this facilitating step seems the most difficult. Some changes—perhaps the most important ones—run counter to the prevailing value system. And yet, ways must be found to demonstrate that the proposed change will *not* violate that system. Failing that, the value system must be modified first. In some cases, time would be better spent on trying to change the value system enough to obtain acceptance of the proposed change than on trying to force acceptance of a proposed change that runs counter to values held dear by a faculty. Inability to perceive this step and to carry it out undoubtedly accounts for widespread failure to achieve truly innovative reform in any schools except those which are newly established and which, therefore, offer the exciting opportunity for the chief administrative officer to recruit new faculty with values consistent with the early innovative plans. If changes are mandated against the prevailing value system, concurrent steps are necessary to precipitate a thoughtful review of that institutional value structure—again by all faculty members.

7. *Change must be perceived as valuable and challenging.* The literature does not contain reports which document failure of reform efforts. If those failures were to be reported, a significant number would include reference to the fact that many faculty in a given school never did see any *reason* to change anything, let alone see any real *value* in the change. In one school where a formal, rigorous program evaluation was attempted in conjunction with the curriculum change, the evaluators asked a sample of faculty members *why* there had been curriculum change—planning to use the rationale for that curriculum change as a set of hypotheses to be tested in the program evaluation design. (e.g., "We wanted to have students make earlier career decisions." Data might then have been collected to test whether the new curriculum did this better than the old one.) The response given to the question, however, was, "The goddamned dean wants us to change the curriculum!" What they were really saying was, "We don't see any value in this curriculum change at all." Now,

again, this step does not mean that all members of the faculty have to perceive the change as valuable at the outset; it means that one of the tasks of the planners is to help faculty review and perceive benefits, value, and challenge in the process.

8. *There must be empathy for those who oppose change.* Those who oppose change—either *per se* or in particular—are still part of the faculty, even if in a small minority. Planners must empathize in order to better plan ways in which to lessen their opposition and minimize their negative influence. All of us have at one time or another found ourselves defending *status quo* in some situation. We would do well to remember the feelings associated with that posture: opponents to our proposals for change are feeling much the same and deserve our thoughtful consideration.

If American medical education is indeed entering a new era of reformation, care must be taken to avoid the pain typically associated with reformation movements. Innovators failing to consider factors opposing change and failing to plan their process steps as carefully as possible will in all probability end up as martyrs—with no assurance that their martyrdom will in any way move medical education closer to their goals. Whatever the *content* of the reformation, the *process* should reflect our best understanding of the dynamics of institutional change.

January 1984

How to Begin Reforming the Curriculum

Howard S. Barrows, M.D.

Many schools have undertaken curricular reforms in the past. They have, on the whole, accomplished little beyond an innovative course or two being added to their curriculum. Many of these attempts have concentrated on adding new content to the curriculum, intensifying the problems of information overload faced today by most medical schools. Other attempts at reform, such as the integration of disciplines using an organ block approach in preclinical years, multiple departmental cooperative efforts in the Introduction of Clinical Medicine, and adding basic science experiences during or after the clinical years, are usually perceived by students and faculty alike as a reshuffling of the same curriculum without any fundamental change in content or delivery. Innovative offerings that feature substantial departures from traditional teaching are usually the result of one or two teachers applying innovative approaches to a small section of the curriculum for which they are totally responsible. When these teachers are replaced, the innovation usually collapses. A few medical schools have developed a small school or separate track with innovative curricula within a traditional school, taking a small subset of students from matriculation to graduation. Although the hope is that they may effect changes in the larger parent organism, survival seems difficult for these transplants for a variety of reasons.

I would suggest that a complex, sophisticated, respected organism such as a traditional medical school, with its well-defined tasks, criteria for success, expected behaviors and reward systems, cannot make any substantial or lasting changes in its educational programs unless there are fundamental changes in educational administration, faculty knowledge and skills, and faculty reward systems. Traditional values and rewards have to be replaced with new ones if any significant or lasting change is to occur. It is on the basis of this assumption that I would suggest the following steps to begin reforming the curriculum of a traditional school. These steps have not been designed with any concern for feasibility from either political or economic viewpoints. They are offered with the belief that a complete and faculty-wide restructuring of educational values and activities is needed to effect any real change.

1. Carry out a faculty-wide retreat of sufficient duration to allow the faculty as a whole to decide on what priority it will assign to the education of men and women for the profession of medicine in relation to the other major tasks of research and patient care. This involves the other major tasks of research and patient care. This involves consideration for what the term "medical school" or "medical college" means. Hopefully the faculty will realize that making the pathway to the career of medicine attractive and enjoyable for talented men and women and producing physicians who will provide better patient care and medical research in the future is both rewarding and of primary importance to the public, the profession of medicine and the country.

2. The faculty, as a whole, should also agree upon the characteristics and competencies expected of their product. What should their students be able to do by the time they are given their M.D. degrees? This statement of expected characteristics should go beyond the limited goals of what facts and concepts students should remember. To develop these stated expectations the faculty might ask the following: Should the medical graduates be:

a. proficient at evaluating patients and making valid decisions about further investigations and care?
b. able to learn on their own, continually assessing their ability to meet the practice challenges confronting them and to remain contemporary in the rapidly evolving fields of medical science and health care delivery?

c. capable of obtaining the latest and best biomedical or clinical information quickly and effectively?
d. able to critically assess the value of information obtained from journals, research, and colleagues?
e. independent thinkers, challenging experts or authority, making decisions when the available and best information is conflicting or inadequate?
f. capable of good interpersonal skills and educational skills with patients, colleagues and other health professionals?
g. concerned about the psychosocial, moral, ethical, or legal aspects of their practice and their role as physicians?

The list can go on and on. Each person on the faculty must honestly and openly express what he or she values. The faculty as a whole must eventually commit themselves in print. In this way the design of a curriculum can be undertaken to produce the characteristics expected by the faculty for graduating students. In addition, teachers will know what needs to be taught and how it should be taught, and valid, relevant assessment tools can be designed to assess the characteristics desired and used. In the same way students will know what is valued and expected to guide their studies and preparation.

3. A system must be established to give teaching faculty encouragement, recognition, and rewards within their own departments and in the school for academic scholarship and excellence in educational service (teaching and evaluation), research, and administration. This system should parallel the reward system for research including promotion, tenure, pay increase, status and perquisites.

4. To provide this scholarship and excellence and achieve the outcomes expected for students, teaching faculty will have to become educated about the science of education and trained for their teaching role. Their knowledge and skills and education should be professionally commensurate with their expertise and skills in patient care and research. They should become prepared for the educational responsibility of student learning. The faculty must be able to go beyond concerns for *what* knowledge they must teach or transfer to medical students and move toward concerns for *how* they must teach in order for the student to learn in

an educational program that must turn out competent physicians at the end. They must be able to evaluate student learning problems when they occur and design individual approaches to help students learn. Over the last few decades, a large body of research in cognitive psychology, educational psychology and in medical education has become available to faculty teachers. This body of knowledge will help them better understand principles of adult learning, organization of useful memory, retention, transfer of skills, the nature of problem-solving skills, the effects of various teaching methods on all of these matters, and how to assess a wide range of competencies. These are all essential for the professionally applied science of medical education. This will require a variety of faculty educational development approaches to be designed and made available such as workshops, short- or long-term fellowships, apprentice experiences, home-study materials, and active educational consultation and support programs.

5. The administration of the curriculum must be a corporate responsibility of the school and not an individual departmental matter. This is the only way to achieve a consistent, organized curriculum that is efficient and effective in meeting the particular school's objectives. Education should be set up as a "horizontal" program that crosses departments and has full responsibility for curricular design and development, faculty and educational resource development, teacher training and assessment, and educational resource development, teacher training and assessment, and maintenance and evaluation of the curriculum. Although such a program under an appropriate administrative hierarchy should be independent of individual medical school departments, it must be responsible to department chairmen as a group through the dean and the executive committee. Departments should provide the appropriate teachers for the educational programs so that assignments can be sensitive to a particular faculty person's other tasks and career development. Each department should also monitor and review the quality of the content delivered in the areas of the curriculum that involve their individual faculty's expertise. The assignment of teachers from the various departments must be a formal process both as to the faculty teacher's commitment of time and the type of teaching activity. Departmental and school consideration of

faculty promotion, tenure, salary increases, etc., must be sensitive to both the teacher's commitment of time to the educational program and his or her excellence in this activity as provided in reports to the chairman.

6. The final step that must be taken in any curricular reform is a realistic, accurate assessment of students against the expected competencies defined by the faculty to evaluate the effectiveness of the curriculum and to assure that a quality product is being graduated. Effective, efficient, and humane patient care requires sophisticated knowledge and skills coupled with a sensitive understanding of people and their problems. The public expects highly professional skills in physicians who have direct responsiblity for the life and well-being of their patients. Although the tools are available for any school to be certain that these skills are present to the degree expected in their graduates, faculty must be willing to step beyond the ease of multiple-choice tests and occasional observations.

Were such steps as these possible, I would have little doubt that the resulting curriculum would be rewarding for both students and faculty. Students would be treated as adults responsible for their own learning using faculty as expert resources in this process similar to graduate education in other fields. The application of sound educational principles to clearly enunciated definitions of expected competencies should lead to learning in functional contexts with students perfecting their reasoning, self-learning, and critical thinking skills as they acquire basic and clinical scientific knowledge.

December 1983

The Ecology of Curriculum Change

James B. Erdmann, Ph.D.

The General Professional Education of the Physician (GPEP) Project of the Association of American Medical Colleges has identified in sharp relief the problems in medical education today that the panelists and those presenting testimony to the panel have agreed need to be addressed. This conference, with its title, *How To Begin Reforming The Medical Curriculum,* would seem to be a logical next step in building upon the GPEP Project and beginning to implement some of the changes implicit in the problems that have been identified. One might ask the question, therefore, where should one start? Reasonable answers might be: 1) where the problem is greatest, or 2) where there is interest among faculty and administration, or 3) where resources are available to attack certain problems, or where some combination of these conditions exist. Any or all of these suggestions seem to be very reasonable and defensible, but they are also the most obvious.

Not so obvious is a dimension of "where to begin" that is easily given insufficient consideration, particularly in the enthusiasm for introducing change. This dimension might be summarized as the environmental impact of the proposed innovation. In short, if one can avoid the bureaucratic connotations associated with the term, it would seem important and useful to prepare an "environmental impact statement" for proposed changes particularly if they are of sufficient significance or magnitude to merit the label "reform."

There are two broad categories of impact that deserve attention, one relating to the characteristics of the strategy or process by which the contemplated change is to be implemented, and the other relating to the effects—intended and unintended— of the change once it is put into place. In the latter case, we are most often concerned about the unintended effects, especially those that are undesirable, and the weighing of those against the benefits that one might realistically expect to achieve once the change is successfully introduced.

Questions that fall into the first category would include:

- What kind of opposition will be developed that cannot be neutralized?
- How much good-will will be used up and unavailable for the future?
- How much resentment will be generated that may imperil future projects?
- How much of a time commitment will be required of collaborators?
- What are the *quid pro quo* obligations assumed to enlist the necessary cooperation?
- What kinds of financial resources will be expended?
- What projects or activities will not be moved as the consequence of the commitment to this effort?

Questions that fall into the second category, the impact of the innovation once in place, include:

- What was there before but is there no longer?
- Who lost what in the process?
- Was it a favorite program of students or faculty?
- How has the balance of power shifted?
- Who is now in control?
- What are the new messages to students and faculty?
- Has the change served to unify or divide the faculty or the student body?
- How does the change relate to the institutional mission?
- What are the long-term financial commitments to keep the program running?
- Will those responsible for the new program be easier or harder to work with?

- Adding this new element to the total picture, what is the overall impression? What kind of balance emerges between the characteristics of the educational program and the characteristics of the end product?

Obviously, the list of questions in both categories could be considerably expanded and not all are applicable to every proposed change. Local factors will also result in different importance being attached to the answers to the various questions. The important consideration seems to be that the process of developing a list and weighing the answers against the realistic expectations of benefits from change becomes an explicit step before change is undertaken.

At this point, it may be useful in exploring the merit of this idea to look at a few problem areas identified in the review of undergraduate medical education for which some change may be appropriate.

Problem: The large number of lecturers assigned to teach in a single course has been observed to be a problem since such a practice has often been associated with poor coordination, redundancy in content and/or lecturers concentrating on their area of interest, with the student overwhelmed by a flood of information that may be quite different from what would be identified as core, basic principles, etc.

Change: A more desirable situation would seem to be a well-coordinated course with the teaching responsibility in the hands of very few with the content focusing primarily on major principles.

Impact Concerns: The focus of interest is not so much on the obvious problems of finding willing and qualified faculty to take on these new responsibilities or even how one handles the reaction of those faculty who may no longer be actively engaged in the teaching program, though the implications of their disengagement from the educational mission of the institution are not so clear. Nor is it too likely to be overlooked that there will be the eventual need to assure the faculty with the heavier teaching load that their involvement is not going to jeopardize their career advancement. These issues are enough part of the change itself so as to require attention if any progress toward implementation is to occur. That is, a systematic impact study may not be needed to bring these concerns to the surface so they can be addressed. A careful look at the educational environment may be necessary though to discover the students' disappointment in no longer being able to come into contact with leading researchers or to learn about developments at the frontiers of medical science. Similarly, the loss of an opportunity to convey the enthusiasm and excitement of those leading researchers for scientific inquiry may result in fewer students giving serious thought to a career in scientific investigation. These concerns are likely to surface only if, for example, all those affected are asked about the impact of such a change on their ambitions and levels of satisfaction.

Problem: The student is treated predominantly as a passive recipient of information, is infrequently challenged to think as opposed to memorizing information and is encouraged to take little responsibility for guiding one's own learning.

Change: The introduction of more small group, problem-based, student-directed learning opportunities is often considered.

Impact Concerns: The criteria by which the student can judge his or her own progress become much more vague.

The depth to which topics should be explored presents a serious dilemma to the students in their attempts to make maximum use of their time.

Uncertainty about one's progress toward satisfying external licensing or certifying requirements increases significantly.

The anxieties and emotional problems of students arising from the preceding concerns grow.

New faculty anxieties involved with their adopting a new and unfamiliar educational role emerge. These concerns include performing a role for which they have had no experience or training, as well as the uncertainty about the impact of their participation on their career development. The lack of experience in evaluating these educational contributions raises concerns about necessary support systems that are important to sustain the new educational format.

At a different level, some may see this new educational style as a move in the direction of upsetting the balance of the educational program even more in the direction of the preparation of academicians or medical scientists. The emphasis of the format would seem to simulate more closely the behavior a scientist should exhibit (i.e., a model of scientific inquiry) than it does the most frequently encountered patient-care situation. The latter situation, some may argue, should be the model for structuring the educational experience if one expects to maximize the transfer from the formal educational setting to the practice setting. Such an educational style is also likely to be expected to be less efficient in accomplishing the necessary objectives and thus leave even less time for concentrating on those aspects of the physician's development which fall under the rubric of the art of medicine. The latter includes skills and habits, it may be argued, which are best formed and refined through repeated practice opportunities.

Problem: A frequently mentioned problem in the area of evaluation has been termed the predominance of the multiple-choice format for testing.

Change: The remedy suggested is a sharp reduction in the use of the multiple-choice format and, in some instances, its total abandonment is recommended.

Impact Concerns: Alternatives to the multiple-choice format usually require significantly more faculty man-hours to score.

Faculty are relatively inexperienced in the creation and use of alternatives. Faculty skills, interest, and support may imply that an entirely new cadre of involved faculty is necessary.

Since the multiple-choice format is perceived to be a measure of straight recall, there may be a problem in the message that it is of little importance.

Student anxiety is sure to increase if opportunities to practice on "board-type" examinations are reduced.

Since multiple-choice formats are particularly suited to measuring the recognition of associations among factors in a patient problem, one must confront the implicit message that that form of information processing is less important to clinical medicine than it once was.

Faculty comfort in the "objectivity" of the scores and the confidence in the precision and impartiality of the scores as a basis for defending judgements of student performance will be seriously decreased. Reluctance to fail students may emerge as a greater problem.

These areas were selected to illustrate the kind of impact

analysis proposed, since they have been identified repeatedly as major areas needing attention in efforts to improve medical education. Surely, the questions and answers will differ for each school and each occasion, and the importance attached to the kinds of negative impact identified will be evaluated differently in each setting.

It is the very nature of environmental impact studies that emphasis is placed on the effect that present changes have on the future balance among all interacting factors. In considering the ecology of the curriculum, this forward-looking perspective on present reform is equally critical. Therefore, any curricular impact statement must include consideration of the directions a specific change will be moving the curriculum and whether that direction is compatible with what we know and expect to be the future demands on the physician. For example, we can predict that advances in computer hardware and software and in medical technology will increasingly be able to assume some of the operations of the physician. We can already see the potential for some of the judgments that physicians make to be assisted by computer simulations of the process.

It would seem incumbent on us to make sure that changes we introduce today are compatible with these developments. Changes that emphasize the aspects of clinical medicine that technology is least suited to handle, such as the functions falling down within the rubric of the art of medicine, might deserve special preference from this perspective. Major concerns have already been voiced about a deficiency in this area. Some would argue that the thrust of medical education should cease competing with the computer but concentrate on maximizing its value in the care of patients. Thus, it would be appropriate to highlight the development of those skills involved in using these emerging resources and technologies.

A significant amount of discussion on reforming or redesigning the educational program has been focused on the value of introducing more problem-solving experiences into the students' learning environment. From one perspective, the development of such a general skill may be the best way to prepare for an uncertain future. From another perspective, it may be important to look specifically at the kind of problem-solving and other experiences we introduce into the curriculum today in the context of whether that is the kind and level of problem-solving or skills we can predict will be needed in the future.

In offering these thoughts, my primary concern is that significant energies, resources, and talent not be devoted now to a massive reform in an educational system that, if accomplished, will be discovered to be out of tune with the realistic needs of society and the development of the profession.

January 1984

Medical Practice in the Future: Current Initiatives and Their Implications for the Physician*

Gordon T. Moore, M.D.

We are, today, at the beginning of a period of unprecedented change in the financing and delivery of medical care in this country. These changes are occuring in response to a number of trends well-documented by multiple authors. These include: a dramatic and compounding rate of increase in the overall costs of medical care in the United States, of which an increasing proportion is borne by government and business; a dramatic increase in the absolute numbers of physicians and other health professionals which will lead to an increasing oversupply of physicians through the turn of the century; the rapid emergence of for-profit medical corporations seeking to deliver both hospital and ambulatory medical services.

These three factors have resulted in several new and powerful initiatives in medical care. First, after years of either hands-off or of interventions which tended to encourage the growth of the medical care industry, both government and business have concluded that cost increases which they bear must be curbed. Their interventions have focused on regulation (diagnostic-related group reimbursement for medicare patients, prospective fixed caps on hospital reimbursement levels); benefit restructuring (reduction in covered benefits which transfer costs of medical

* Dr. Moore's paper, submitted at the time of the conference, was not among the original group of protagonist papers. However, it introduces several important themes relevant to discussions of the preparation of students for the practice of medicine in the future. Because these themes are central to many of the conference discussions, the paper has been included here.

care increasingly to consumers, attempts to reduce the before-tax status of medical insurance premiums); public exhortation (activities of individual businesses, local business coalitions, and the national business counsel); and attempts to stimulate competitive delivery systems competing to reduce costs to consumers and third-party payers (the HMO Act of 1973, increased business support for HMO alternatives for their employees).

The shape of the national response to these initiatives is gradually emerging. The rapid growth of pre-paid health care delivery systems which began approximately five years ago continues to accelerate (upwards of 18 to 20% increases in national membership over the past year) and the for-profit sector is one of the most vigorous components of this growth. Second, intense competition among and between components of the delivery system is occurring, with new variations of delivery and finance emerging rapidly. Among these variations are competition among physicians and between physicians and hospitals for patients and patient revenues, the diversification of hospitals into new revenue-stimulating ventures, the development of non-hospital systems to compete with emergency rooms and hospital-based surgery, a beginning of redistribution of physicians into suburban and ex-urban areas, and the development of physician and institutional consortia designed to market reduced-cost packages to insurers and businesses.

These trends are dramatic and, as other authors have pointed out, physicians will increasingly practice in bureaucratic business organizations and will be reimbursed prospectively, either by salaried arrangements or by receipt of a capitation for patients whose care they assume. Fee-for-service medicine will dramatically decrease in the future.

While dramatic, these trends are likely to have more effect on the financing and the business culture of medicine than on the practice of medicine itself. However, emerging from these early trends are three major themes which will more significantly affect the manner in which physicians practice medicine in the future. First among these is the change in the nature of services which physicians will be delivering. In the circumstances of increased numbers of physicians, business- and for-profit-oriented delivery mechanisms, and a relative stricturing of the third-party dollars flowing in to cover illness care, new markets for medical services will develop. Many of these will be adaptive responses to changes in financing, as has occurred historically. Major growth will occur in newly-defined services which have not been actively developed in the past. These will include a significantly expanded home care industry; vastly increased levels of consumer-oriented services such as extended hours and house calls, emphasizing greater access and convenience; and "wellness" services focusing on health behaviors, psychological or counseling services, prevention and screening for disease. A push for new markets will force physician adaptation into areas of medical care long ago delegated to other health professionals, into services abandoned in the past, and into new services when consumers will pay for them. A significant number of physicians will be called upon to carry out these activities with relatively little prior training or experience, and a multitude of entrepreneurial ventures will develop to plan, organize, finance, and re-train physicians to enable the delivery of these services. The very nature of what we currently consider to be the purview of the physician in delivering medical care will change dramatically, even though the illness-oriented and scientifically and technically-based medical care system as we now know it will continue.

A second major alteration in the way physicians practice will occur because of the need to allocate increasingly scarce medical resources. With decreased funding, high cost medical diagnosis and procedures will become decreasingly available. While the last twenty years have marked an unprecedented increase in accessibility of Americans to medical care, the financially open-ended system which supported this is ending. Increasing sectors of the American population will become financially disenfranchised, but the entire population, in addition, will be competing for more limited resources in which the major allocation decisions will be made by physicians. As in England, most of these allocation decisions will be made at the local level, in hospitals and offices, by individual physicians dealing with individual patients. This trend will require physicians to become sophisticated about the costs of diagnosis and treatment, about optimal decision-making pathways, and about priority-setting around the use of limited facilities, tests, equipment and therapies. An increased need to learn negotiating strategies and a heightened pressure on the physician's sense of moral and ethical responsibility to his patients will increase the day-to-day strain and conflict of being a physician. The relatively easy relationship between physician and patient pursuing an unconstrained diagnostic and therapeutic plan will be replaced by the physician acting as broker for the patient. Patient financial capacity, likely clinical outcomes, personal persuasion, and values and beliefs of the physician will enter significantly into the access of patients to potentially needed or desired medical services.

The third, and most profound, change will pit the physician against his patient. The control of medical care costs will ultimately fall on physicians. Although other alternatives exist, the most powerful themes emerging from the responses to achieve cost-control have been those in which expenditures are set prospectively, and physicians, hospitals or other organized delivery mechanisms must care for patients within these financial caps. HMOs have long known, hospitals are discovering and capitated networks of physicians are quickly adapting to systems in which physicians are given financial incentive, direct or indirect, to deliver services within a budgeted amoung. The more direct the financial reward to the physician for reducing expenditures for consultations, tests, procedures and therapies, the greater the financial benefit is to the delivery system and to the physician. Although the incentive for this is perhaps greater in for-profit systems, no system which is prospectively reimbursed and operates within a fixed budget will avoid this conflict between patient and physician. When the conflict is direct and personal, as in the case of physicians who receive a capitation for each patient and then are expected to pay for needed medical services for their patients out of this capitation (keeping as income that which is left over), the conflict is real and powerful. In this setting, the physician directly profits from the reduction of services which his patients might well, today, expect to receive; this will put severe strain on the trust and relationship between doctor and patient.

Against this background, one can examine the likely impact and outcome of this change. As Paul Starr so elegantly points out, the profession of medicine has historically given physicians, themselves, the right and privilege of setting and guarding its own standards of professionalism and quality.* For the first time in the history of medicine, physicians have very significant life-prolonging services to give to patients and the financing and delivery systems are moving to benefit the physician for withholding these services. This restructuring of the dynamics of the relationship between patient and physician will make it increasingly likely that standards and quality assessment will become an audit function external to the profession. It is highly likely that external review stimulated by government, business and consumer groups will increasingly demand evidence of quality, explicit review of the physician's decision pathway and the delivery system. In this setting, quality assurance and quality audit, which have developed only to a meager level in the past, will accelerate as independent measures of the work which physicians do. Physicians and the delivery systems in which they practice can expect increasingly powerful and effective review of the work that they do in the future.

June 1984

---

* P. Starr, *The Social Transformation of American Medicine* (New York: Basic Books, 1982).

Some Thoughts on Curriculum Change in Medical Education

Vic R. Neufeld, M.D.

How can a medical school change its curriculum? In this essay, I shall suggest four sets of considerations, all of which influence the answer to this question. These considerations are:

1. The context in which medical education occurs.
2. The strategies available to an individual medical school.
3. The influence of organizations, local and national.
4. The role of individuality.

The Context

The ultimate purpose of medical education is the preparation of physicians who will contribute to easing the "burden of illness" and maintaining the health status of the population. Mostly, this will be done through the provision of health care to individual patients. If this statement of purpose is acceptable, it is important to recognize the following facts about health and health care.

- The major determinants of human health are where we live and how we live, and not the health care we receive; perhaps more important than the "health care delivery system" are other factors such as nutrition, sanitation, transportation, housing and employment. For example, there is a clear relationship between poverty and health status.

- Using common indicators of health (such as life expectancy and infant mortality), there has been relatively little change in the health status of our society in the last decade or more; nevertheless, the costs of health care have risen steadily.
- Given the above, the main influence of the health care system and of the health professionals who provide care is on the quality of life of individuals who are ill or who think they are ill.
- Within the health care system, physicians are only one of the "actors"; others are health administrators, allied health professionals, government officers, and private health and insurance agencies. There is also a vast "para-health network" of individuals and organizations who provide health care.
- Many of the interventions used by physicians have not been scientifically demonstrated to improve health outcomes; and some do more harm than good.
- There is an inappropriately long delay between the time that valid knowledge (which would improve health outcomes) is published, and when it is actually put into practice by physicians.

Despite the above, our society has granted physicians the official responsibility to determine the absence or presence of illness. Individual physicians have a major impact on the effectiveness and efficiency with which health-care interventions are used to affect the quality of life.

The medical school, through its admissions process and its curriculum, represents the gateway through which individuals pass on their way to becoming licensed practitioners. The contextual statements listed above should be strongly considered when stating the competencies to be demonstrated by medical school graduates—the "end product" of the general professional education which is provided by the medical school.

The Individual Medical School

Far from being a helpless giant, each medical school has within its power the ability to make substantial changes in its education program. However, certain conditions need to be in place in order for changes to occur. These include the following:

1. A statement of educational purpose:
   This is primarily a description of the "end product" which the medical curriculum is designed to produce (an example of such a statement can be found in the "General Objectives: M.D. Program, McMaster University," included as an addendum to this paper). The statement may include the strategies which a faculty intends to use in deploying its resources efficiently; it may even mention that individual faculty members should expect to perform their educational roles with enjoyment and satisfaction.
2. A corporate sense:
   A medical education program represents only one of the functions of a medical school. It is critical that the "community of scholars" in a medical school has a sense of the relative priorities of institutional goals. The sub-units (such as departments) can be seen as repositories of expertise, contributing not only to individual and departmental goals, but to the corporate mission.
3. A system of faculty incentives and rewards:
   Although this will vary from one institution to another, the following elements seem to be essential:
   a. The recognition that there are various educational roles which can be defined; an individual faculty member may be more suited to one task than another.
   b. A clear promotions and tenure statement that educational contributions are recognized as essential; this should be validated by actual institutional behavior.
   c. At least a quantitative record of an individual faculty member's contribution to education. For some key roles, additional qualitative information should be obtained.
   d. New faculty members require an orientation to the objectives and methods of the curriculum.
4. A cadre of educational leaders:
   In order to keep the educational mission clearly in the view of the faculty, it is essential that a few individuals make the education program their primary task. The task includes both short- and long-range planning, efficient implementation, and ongoing curriculum review. This leadership function can be enhanced by special training programs, emphasizing principles of learning,

evaluation, and organizational management.

5. A long-range view:

It must be recognized that human behavior (usually) changes slowly and in small steps. Hence, a curriculum change may take several years to develop and implement. The educational leadership needs to be clear and firm about long-range objectives, but flexible about the timing and methods to achieve them. A sense of opportunism is helpful, when an unexpected situation can be used to move the educational enterprise forward.

Inter-Institutional and National Influences

There are other influences originating from outside a medical school. The planners of a curriculum can ignore them; they can recognize them and adapt; or they can devote some energies into shaping the entity which is affecting the medical school. Some of these influences are listed below, with a comment on what an individual medical school might do about them.

1. Multi-institutional Health Care Systems:

It has been predicted that these corporate entities, in a price-competitive environment, will increasingly influence the nature of medical education. Medical schools should anticipate the kind of physician that can provide positive future leadership in these private health care systems.

2. The Accreditation System:

The nation's medical schools have at least "half shares" in the current accreditation system. It should be possible to propose a change in the accreditation process which would direct institutional self-study to include such questions as these:

a. What is your intended "end-product"?

b. What is the evidence that you are producing this product?

c. Are the teaching/learning processes optimally arranged to achieve this goal?

d. Do your students enjoy their medical education?

3. The Licensing System:

The boards of the national examination agencies (specifically the NBME) are comprised largely by faculty members of medical schools. Rather than excessive and useless "scapegoating" of the NBME, it would be useful to join in discussion with the agency to accelerate the development of evaluation tools which test important competencies and to minimize the abuse of NBME test results.

4. Networks:

There is considerable benefit in the development of informal networks of institutions with similar interests in medical education. These groups could focus on specific innovations over a defined time period with the outcome of producing materials (manuals, learning resources, reports) which will benefit the medical education community.

5. Funding for Educational Research:

The research base on the process and outcomes of medical education is deficient. Assumptions about educational practice remain untested. Many important questions either have not been explored or the available data are quite old. Major initiatives are needed to strengthen research and develop in medical education, given the continuing interest of our society in matters of health and illness. It surely cannot be outside our collective imagination and capability to create the arrangements for productive research in this field.

The Role of Individuality

We need to remember that in the final analysis, learning is an individual affair. While no doubt planned arrangements (such as a medical school curriculum) have some influence on the making of a doctor, these are not the only determinants. Frequently, an unplanned, unanticipated situation may have a profound effect on the shaping of a medical student; examples include a particular contact with a patient, a personal experience, or time spent with a gifted teacher.

A long-lasting impact can be made by an individual clinical teacher who shows a consistent example in his own work of honesty, compassion, more interest in good questions than pat answers, and an unbridled enjoyment of the practice of medicine.

November 1983

Addendum: General Objectives, M.D. Program, McMaster University*

The aim of the M.D. Program is to provide students with a general professional education as physicians. The program enables students to build on previous education and experience, using available learning resources and opportunities. The competencies achieved by graduates will qualify them to proceed to further postgraduate training. While most graduates will be involved directly with the care of individual patients, it is expected that some will choose careers concerned with the health of populations and the development of new knowledge.

The overriding objective to be achieved is the demonstrated ability to identify, analyse and manage clinical problems in order to provide effective, efficient and humane patient care.

Enabling objectives consisting of knowledge, skills and personal qualities to be achieved are the following:

Knowledge:

1. To acquire and put into practice concepts and information required to understand and manage health care problems. The study of human structure, function and behavior will be guided by an analysis of the determinants of health and illness. A spectrum of factors will be considered in both the external and internal environments of individuals, when deciding on preventive, therapeutic, rehabilitative and supportive management.

* Dr. Neufeld submitted with his paper these commencement objectives specified by the McMaster University faculty.

Skills:

To acquire and use the following skills:

2. Critical Appraisal Skills: The application of certain rules of evidence of clinical, investigational and published data in order to determine their validity and applicability.

3. Clinical Skills: The ability to acquire, interpret, synthesize and record clinical information in managing the health problems of patients, considering their physical, social and emotional function. Included is the use of the clinical reasoning process.

4. Self-Directed Learning Skills: The ability to identify areas of deficiency in one's own performance, find appropriate educational resources, evaluate personal learning progress, and use new knowledge and skills in the care of patients.

Personal Qualities:

5. To recognize, develop and maintain the personal qualities required for a career as a health professional. Acquiring the authority to intervene in the lives of patients carries with it the obligation to act responsibly:

   a. Toward oneself: to recognize and acknowledge personal assets, emotional reactions, and limitations, in one's own knowledge, skills and attitudes, and to do something about them.

   b. Toward patients and their families: to be able, under appropriate supervision, to take responsibility for the assessment and care of patients and their families.

   c. Toward colleagues: to contribute to productive communication and cooperation among colleagues engaged in learning, research or health care.

   d. Toward the community: to contribute to the maintenance and improvement of the health of the general population.

Possible Approaches for Improving Medical Education

Parker A. Small, Jr., M.D., Peter M. Small, and Parker A. Small, III

Introduction

One of us (PAS, Jr.) was asked to propose some concrete suggestions by which classic medical schools could improve their medical education programs. In order to do this, aid was sought from a medical student (PMS) and a graduate student of business (PAS III) involved in a case study approach to learning. This paper is divided into three major sections. The first summarizes major problems we perceive to exist with basic science and clinical education at many medical schools. The second part suggests possible changes that might help alleviate the perceived problems, and the third part suggests possible strategies for introducing the necessary changes.

Problems with Medical Education circa 1984

This section will first address problems with basic science education and then problems with clinical education, although the separation of the two domains is itself one of the problems. It is our view that basic science education has serious flaws that desperately need improvement and that clinical education could profit from some "fine tuning."

A. Problems with Basic Science Medical Education
1. *Loss of contact between students and faculty.*

Basic science medical education two to three decades ago had much more laboratory time, fewer lectures and smaller classes. This meant that faculty and students got to know each other, especially during the laboratory exercises. Unfortunately, many of the exercises were of questionable relevance or value and hence were eliminated over the last two decades. Equally unfortunate, they were often replaced by additional lectures and their associated factual load. Hence today, at many schools, the average student may go through the first two years of medical school without getting to know a single faculty member, and the average basic science faculty member will know the names of fewer than five medical students, much less know them as human beings. This lack of communication has enabled the basic science curriculum to evolve further toward a sometimes dehumanizing, fact-filled feat of memorization rather than a stimulating and enjoyable opportunity to understand human biology. This unfortunate evolution of the curriculum stems in part from the lack of communication between students and faculty. This lack has even contributed to mutual antagonism between some basic science faculty and some medical students at a few schools.

2. *Overemphasis on facts and inadequate emphasis on other critical aspects of education.*

It is an interesting dichotomy that most basic science faculty pride themselves on their ability to teach their graduate students how to acquire and manipulate data but focus on giving medical students only facts and concepts. The loss of laboratories also led to a decrease of data analysis skills and technical skills in the curriculum. If this focus on facts was ever justified, it will be progressively less defensible as our knowledge base grows and our data retrieval capabilities are further augmented by computers. In addition to the limited cognitive goals, there is almost no focus on interpersonal skills in most basic science education.

3. *The information that is learned in basic science is often learned in a context unrelated to clinical problems.*

There is a growing evidence that if material is learned in one context and used in another, much less information will be transferred than if learned in the context of its subsequent use. More recent research suggests that students must be informed that there is a relationship between the information and the problem for them to subsequently be able to use the information to solve the problem.* Relevance is not just a battle cry of the '60s and a motivator. It seems to be an essential component of useful learning.

4. *Evaluation by multiple-choice questions (MCQs)*.

A review of the microbiology final exams of about two dozen medical schools and a subset of the NBME test item library of MCQs leads to the conclusion that over 90% require only recognition of isolated facts. Few questions require data analysis and fewer yet require any problem-solving. Since the evaluation system drives the educational system, students are motivated primarily to memorize facts so that they can be recognized on MCQ tests. Large class size and other forces have led to MCQs being the preponderant, and in some courses the sole, evaluation technique. This has led to even more focus on isolated facts and misled students in the pursuit of quick answers rather than the investigative processes. They are conditioned to blindly accept the faculty's word rather than develop the critical analysis necessary to be good physicians. Understanding, reasoning, and the use of other higher cognitive functions are counterproductive if such actions take time away from memorizing additional facts. This is not to say that MCQs have no place in medical education—they do! However, the MCQs must measure higher cognitive function and MCQs must be only part of the evaluation system.

B. Problems with Clinical Medical Education

Clinical education is fundamentally an apprenticeship experience and as such its quality is proportional to the quality of the mentor and the appropriateness of the feedback.

1. *Goal.*

Clinical education must help the student to further develop his or her problem-solving skills. This requires an emphasis on data-acquisition skills and data-analysis skills and their

---

* G.A. Perfetto, J.D. Bransford and J.J. Franks, "Constraints on Access in a Problem-Solving Context." *Memory and Cognition 11* (1983):24-51.

use to elucidate the pathophysiologic processes taking place in their patients. It is not the time to develop an encyclopedic knowledge of specific disease entities.

2. *Mentor selection.*

At many medical schools there are tremendous differences from service to service and even month to month on the same service in the quantity and quality of clinical teaching. Theoretically, clinical education is primarily the duty of the attending physician. However, due to the multiplicity of faculty responsibilities (many of which are perceived as having higher priorities), the teaching of medical students is frequently delegated to the house staff. More attention should be given to identifying those clinicians who are most interested in teaching and assigning them to clearly defined teaching roles with less responsibility in other areas.

3. *Feedback and evaluation.*

Clearer definitions of objectives and more precise measures of their attainment are required. The student who happily does the "scut" and is always available may be more highly rewarded by hard-pressed house staff than the student who spends more time out of sight but with patients and books.

Desired Changes in Medical Education

These proposed changes are divided into curriculum changes and instructional changes. Our proposals relative to the former are more radical and less realistic, but this is consistent with our belief that curriculum changes are less worthwhile and lasting than instructional changes.

A. Curriculum Changes

The following two-part proposal for curriculum change is one of many possible approaches. It is intended to be illustrative and provocative, certainly not optimal or exhaustive. The essence of the proposal is to transfer learning of basic science from the passive lecture mode to an active problem-solving mode. The radical nature of the proposal may be shocking to some readers.

1. *Drastically condense classic basic science.*

We suggest that the classic first two years of medical school be condensed by three quarters to no more than one semester. The major goal is to create a situation where there is no time to focus on facts, only time to get a quick overview of each discipline and to understand how to access information within those disciplines. We would limit the number of lectures to two per day to help prevent the faculty from using the approach of "talk four times faster to make up for the time cut." We would stress appropriate labs, discussion groups and other approaches for most of the instructional time. Ideally basic science faculty should realize their responsibility for teaching not just facts, but data acquisition, data analysis, technical and even interpersonal skills.

There is a subset of faculty who are primarily involved in research and graduate education and who have little interest in medical education. We believe this group should be involved in special projects such as independent study projects for individual medical students but not in the regular curriculum unless they express a desire for such involvement.* This group of faculty is contributing to the institution in other ways and should not be forced to contribute directly to medical education.

2. *Preclinical patient-oriented problem-solving.*

The remaining three semesters of basic science would be predominantly devoted to solving clinical problems. These problems would be presented in an organized way but in a variety of formats to ensure that the student will have to identify and utilize appropriate basic science concepts from all disciplines to successfully solve progressively more complex clinical problems. During this phase we would advocate the use of PBLM formats similar to those developed at SIU, POPS formats like those developed at Florida, CPC-format tutorials based on case histories. We would encourage experimentation with a wide variety of formats. Much is to be learned from an evaluation of whole class problem-solving formats similar to those utilized at the Harvard Business School for over 50 years. The basic idea is to provide students with a stimulus to identify for themselves the data necessary to understand clinical problems, to seek the data in

---

* See R.G. Petersdorf, "Sounding Board: Is the Establishment Defensible?" *NEJM* 309 (1983):1053.

texts, archival literature and from peers and faculty, and then to utilize the data in the solution/understanding of the problem. All of this would, however, take place without the human, temporal and financial constraints placed on learning related to real patients. This program would require a carefully trained subset of faculty consisting of both basic and clinical scientists.

There would be a need for different schools to share their formats, problems and experiences so that the medical schools of the nation could all profit from their combined trials and errors. During this phase of the curriculum, students would also be learning how to take a history and do a physical exam.

B. Instructional Changes

1. *Use of simulated patients and patient instructors.*

The use of simulated patients and patient instructors (SP/PI) for the teaching of history taking and physical diagnosis is a powerful innovation that is being fostered by SIU. A national network for the training and exchange of such people would lead to a major advance in medical education. SIU should take the lead in establishing this national resource.

2. *Evaluation.*

Appropriate evaluation is essential for optimal function of any system. The flawed evaluation system in medical education is partly responsible for our current problems. As stated earlier, fact recognition is all that is currently tested in Parts I and II of the NBME examinations. Reform is urgent. The time per MCQ must be increased so that higher cognitive functions can be tested. This requires a reduction in the number of MCQs and that, in turn, requires an acceptance on the part of medical schools and licensing bodies that applicants' scores will not be reported for each separate discipline, but only for basic and clinical science. This results from the necessity of having a large enough number of test items to give a statistically reliable score. The performance of a school's class could still be evaluated in each discipline. The second NBME change that seems urgent is for there to be increased experimentation with non-MCQ formats. Simulated patients and patient evaluators seem to be an exciting possibility.

At the medical school level clinical evaluation also should involve SP/PI. Historically, our inability to identify a good physician has led to our inability to be able to identify good medical education. It has been analogous to trying to isolate an enzyme without an assay for the enzyme. SP/PIs provide a way of assaying most of the many skills necessary for being a good doctor. This then provides the tool for a giant step forward in medical education.

Other powerful new tools that should be used in medical schools include the triple jump exam wherein students are presented a problem and encouraged to go as far toward the solution as their knowledge base permits, but to also identify the necessary additional knowledge required. They then are given a few hours to obtain that information and then are examined again. Thus one can evaluate not just their data base and data-management skills, but their data-acquisition skills, as well.

Strategies for Instituting Change

Although we have identified some specific changes and even suggested a specific curriculum in the previous sections, the specific changes that are optimal or even possible will vary from school to school. It is undoubtedly more important for each medical school to develop a process that will promote and sustain evolution of the instructional program than to institute any specific change. The purpose of this section is to suggest possible steps in the development of that process.

A. Identify the Goals of the Medical Education Program

As with any undertaking, the first step is to identify the goal or goals. One problem is that many faculty do not understand the importance of clear, measurable goals for medical education. These goals must be stated in a way such that their attainment can be evaluated. Some perceive the creation of such goals to be a waste of time while others have such a narrow view of their own role within the medical school that they have difficulty conceptualizing broader goals. It is essential, however, to get agreement among the faculty, especially chairpeople and other opinion leaders, as to the goals of the medical education program.

One way to accomplish this is to have each faculty member write their own goals for the program and then share these usually diverse documents with the group. This has the advantage of actively involving the participants but can have disadvantage of locking some people into a position of defending their own ideas "to the death." A second approach is to get the faculty to respond to comparable documents from other institutions. In either case, the goal is for the faculty to produce a written document which clearly identifies the goals and does so in a way that will subsequently promote data collection to establish whether the goals are being met.

B. Determine Faculty and Student Perceptions of How Well the Goals Are Being Met

It is very difficult to impose change on a system that is perceived by most of those involved to be functioning well. An early step must therefore be to determine whether the faculty and students perceive problems. This can be done by having them match the institutional goals with their own perception of what is taking place. One possible approach is to carefully construct a questionnaire which includes the institutional goals. The faculty and students also must be alerted to the role the goals and questionnaire are to play in the evolution of the instructional program.

C. Establish Mechanisms Whereby Faculty and Students can Exchange Views of Possible Problems

Based on the response of the faculty and students to the questionnaire or whatever other mechanism is used, the next step is to create an environment which will promote an exchange among the faculty and students. One possible approach is to have a workshop and invite faculty whose responses to the questionnaire were most insightful. The goal of this activity is for the group to reach a consensus as to whether there are problems, and if so, what those problems are.

D. Create an Institutional Plan for Improving Medical Education

Once a reasonable consensus has been achieved as to existing problems, the next step is to redistribute the interested faculty and perhaps students into a new set of small groups and to charge these new groups with developing a proposal to improve the educational program. The goal is to create a system with adequate feedback and rewards so that the educational system will continue to evolve toward more complete attainment of the goals. It is essential that the proposal include contingencies for rewarding faculty that contribute to medical education. As noted earlier, at some institutions young faculty who devote too much time to medical education jeopardize their careers. New rewards must be found to balance the rewards for research and patient care. Classically, teachers get their most powerful reward from seeing their students learn and grow. The system must evolve back to a state where basic science students and faculty know each other well enough so that the faculty can directly observe the students' growth. However, additional rewards must also be found. Some possible examples of such rewards might be that each class of medical students be given a substantial amount of money to divide as the students see fit among their teachers. This would promote the development of an evaluation system of faculty by students, and would enhance the student's interest in contributing to that evaluation system. Because faculty sometimes appreciate different values in teachers, course directors should also be given a similar amount of money to distribute to the faculty. One of the greatest administrative challenges is to create appropriate contingencies for the faculty.

Summary

There is a growing awareness that medical education has some major problems. It is essential that our medical education leaders mobilize the institutional resources so that each medical school can 1) establish goals against which progress can be measured, 2) identify the problems, 3) establish a process to improve the system, and 4) establish feedback mechanisms which will sustain an ongoing evolution toward more complete achievement of the educational goals of the institution. Some radical possibilities are discussed, including 1) a drastic shortening of the classic, lecture dependent, basic science curriculum and a substitution of a period wherein students are actively involved in learning basic science and applying it to clinical problems and 2) giving funds to students for them to use to directly reward teaching faculty. We hope that these purposefully provocative proposals will help to stimulate discussions which in turn will help to solve some of the problems.

The fundamental problem is that there is a feedback system to identify productivity for research and patient care but not for education. Although imperfect, the published papers and research grants of an individual or department provide a measure of research productivity. The number of patients seen and patient fee income provide a measure of the quantity of patient care. The interaction of faculty, house staff and students provides a mechanism for maintenance of quality of care. In contrast, the number of medical students in most classes is constant and not dependent on the quality of the course. More important, there is no adequate measure of the quality of the medical education received by the students nor of the skill of any specific graduate. NBME examinations currently measure only recall of specific facts, and this is not an adequate measure of the skills necessary to be a good physician. Given the feedback for research and patient care and the lack of comparable feedback for education, it is predictable that faculty effort devoted to education will decrease. Until a more adequate feedback system for medical education is developed, serious problems with the system will persist.

January 1984

Addendum: The Introduction of "Clinical Problem-Solving Days" into the Basic Science Curriculum

Parker A. Small, Jr., M.D.

Having proposed some purposefully provocative and not necessarily realistic suggestions, we would now like to put forth a more realistic approach to the introduction of clinically relevant problem solving into a classic basic science curriculum.

A major challenge for medical faculty is to help students to better integrate their basic science knowledge into the clinical framework in which they will be working. One way of looking at the basic science/clinical science division within medical education is to contrast the synthetic or bottom-up approach of the traditional basic scientist with the degradative or top-down approach of the clinician. By synthetic or bottom-up, we mean that basic scientists like to teach from simple to complex. For example, they like to start with amino acids, move on the synthesis of antibody molecules, then discuss the function of the antibodies and finally relate that to host defense. In contrast to this, the degradative or top-down approach of the clinician must begin with a patient, e.g., one who suffers from recurrent infections. The clinician proceeds to evaluate several broad categories of host defense mechanisms and investigates antibody function and specific details of the antibody system. This brings into focus the basic science that he knows. The medical student must be able to combine the two approaches. With the classic curriculum the student often spends 1 to 2 years with the bottom-up approach before he begins to look at things from the other direction. The challenge then is to help the student to frequently flip back and forth between the bottom-up and top-down approaches.

In order to accomplish this we propose the introduction of "Clinical Problem-Solving Days" into the basic science curriculum.

Let us begin by describing a typical day. Those of you who have had the opportunity to visit SIU and observe Howard Barrows teaching will immediately recognize that we are describing the process that he uses and you will also recognize its resemblance to the triple jump exam used at McMaster. The day has 3 parts: 1) problem presentation and identification of learning issues, 2) independent study time, and 3) synthesis and evaluation time. Part one would take about an hour and begin with the presentation of a clinical problem to groups of 4 to 6 medical students. On different days faculty would use different formats to present the problem. For example, early in the students' career, printed CPC formats, similar to those used at New Mexico, would enable students to begin to formulate hypotheses, relate clinical data with basic science concepts and identify learning issues. Later, when students have more understanding of the process of taking a history and doing a physical exam, other formats that enable students to practice data acquisition skills could be utilized. These formats would include PBLMs, faculty supplying the information that the patient would have given, simulated patients and perhaps even an occasional real patient. By the end of part one, students should have developed a data base, formulated a number of hypotheses as to the nature of the problem, identified for themselves a group of issues about which they need to learn more and assigned these learning issues to specific group members.

Part two consists of each group member going to the library and/or other resources to learn about his or her learning issues. This phase of the Problem-Solving Day should take 4 to 6 hours. For Phase Three, the faculty and students reconvene for a one- to two-hour session wherein the students teach each other what they have learned, reformulate their understanding of the clinical problem, and finally evaluate their own performances. It is important to keep the goal of this process in mind. It is *not* to arrive at a correct diagnosis, but rather to practice hypothesis generation, data acquisition, data analysis and interpersonal skills and in so doing to utilize in a top-down manner the basic science information they had been learning in a bottom-up fashion.

Picking a day as an educational period has the advantage that the amount of total curriculum time can evolve. For example, such problem solving days could initially be introduced at a frequency of one per month and if found to be worthwhile, increased in subsequent years to one per week or even more. The remaining time can continue to be used in the usual fashion. The selection of a day, rather than a longer period of time, is to constrain the process so that students will not get so caught up in learning about the patients' problems that they might take time from their classic studies and not do as well in them. Limiting the process to one day and involving the entire class in it should keep the process from punishing the most inquisitive students.

The role of the faculty is to facilitate the process and not to be sources of information. We suggest that two faculty be assigned to each group of students. By having two faculty they can keep each other from turning the session into a series of mini-lectures. It also provides "on-the-job training" for less experienced teachers since they can be matched with experienced group leaders and thus a larger group of trained faculty can be created. If one faculty member comes from basic science and the other from clinical science there is the further advantage that the basic science faculty person will develop more breadth and a better understanding of how basic science fits into clinical medicine, while the clinical faculty may develop more in-depth knowledge and perhaps a more critical approach to data analysis.

In summary, the "Clinical Problem-Solving Day" format permits the non-disruptive introduction of new teaching methods into traditional curricula.

June 1984

The Oliver Wendell Holmes Society:
A New Pathway to General Medical Education at Harvard Medical School*

Introduction

In June of 1983, the Harvard Faculty of Medicine approved the overall goals and general outline of an experimental pathway for the general education of physicians, a new academic society, to be called the Oliver Wendell Holmes Society. This New Pathway will admit 25 students from our entering class of 165, beginning in September 1985. The project has called for a serious examination of medical education from a fresh vantage point, beginning with our most fundamental assumptions about the attitudes, skills and knowledge that physicians today and tomorrow must strive to possess. It has been our goal to think, from the ground up, about the entire span of general medical education, and to give as much attention to *how* medicine is learned as to *what* that learning should entail.

Any assessment of the ways best to prepare physicians to bring medicine into the twenty-first century must begin with an analysis of changing conditions, both within medicine and in the society physicians serve. In the 1980s, change is more dramatically apparent in medicine than in any other professional sector of American society. Within the last decades, advances in the pace of scientific and technological discovery have profoundly altered the body of medical knowledge. Developments in the sciences that bear on human health and disease have led to entirely new understandings of the workings of the human body—

---

* Excerpted from a progress report submitted to the Harvard Medical Curriculum Committee in May 1984. Contributed as a protagonist paper for the Macy/SIU conference by Daniel C. Tosteson, M.D., Dean, Harvard Medical School. This report represents ongoing discussions of the Harvard New Pathway program.

with implications for our very sense of what it is to be human. Recent advances, particularly in molecular and cell biology, immunology and neurobiology, have opened new paths to preventive, diagnostic and curative strategies of astonishing power and subtlety.

The very extent and sophistication of our knowledge have prompted basic changes in the organization of medical research and practice. Hence, as the fraction of the total spectrum of knowledge that can be mastered by the individual continually diminishes, the number of medical specialties has grown, yielding an increasingly fragmented medical practice. The many new applications of technology to medicine, while greatly enhancing our diagnostic and therapeutic power, have introduced a new contradiction for practitioners: the incongruity between their role as expert technologists, on the one hand, and as counselors and guides, on the other. Lewis Thomas reminds us that:

> . . . touching with the naked ear was one of the great advances in the history of medicine. Once it was learned that the heart and lungs made sounds of their own, and that the sounds were sometimes useful for diagnosis, physicians placed an ear over the heart, and over areas on the front and back of the chest, and listened. It is hard to imagine a friendlier gesture, a more intimate signal of personal concern and affection, than these close bowed heads affixed to the skin. The stethoscope was invented in the nineteenth century, vastly enhancing the acoustics of the thorax, but removing the physician a certain distance from his patient. . . . Today, the doctor can perform a great many of his most essential tasks from his office in another building without ever seeing the patient.*

No less challenging are the changes originating outside of medicine. The public and private demand for containment of medical and hospital costs, and the resultant shift from cost reimbursement to prospective budgeting in hospitals, have so altered the economics of health care that medical and financial incentives are no longer congruent, but conflicting. Advancements in the information sciences are dramatically altering the ways in which physicians practice their craft, providing us with new ways to solve old problems, and reshaping the very environment in which medicine is learned and practiced. An increasingly in-

---

* L. Thomas, *The Youngest Science* (New York: The Viking Press, 1983).

formed and concerned American public is challenging providers of health care to establish more humane methods of clinical practice—to create a more equal partnership between physicians and patients, and to encourage patients to assume primary responsibility for their own health care and treatment.

Alongside these far-reaching developments that are changing the shape of medicine from within and without are aspects of the physician's relationship to the sick and suffering that remain relatively unchanging. Time-honored skills of caring and responsibility have always been part of the physician's repertoire. The experience of illness, unique for each individual, has always presented a vast array of intangible elements that the physician must strive to understand in an encounter with a patient. Many different factors are entangled in the problems patients present, making causal inferences extremely difficult, and no predictive measures can fully anticipate the course and outcome of any single medical encounter. Paradoxically, despite the revolution in the sciences and technologies underlying medicine, physicians continue—as they always will—to practice their art in the midst of uncertainty.

There is, in short, a growing tension between the changing and unchanging faces of medicine. Today, those responsible for the education of physicians must confront this paradox. We must help future physicians to address *both* the ever-changing, ever-broadening and deepening mass of knowledge bearing on the etiology and cure of disease *and* the relatively unchanging aspects of medicine that are founded on the relationship of an individual physician to an individual patient.

There will always be a need to scrutinize and assess established patterns in medical education for their effectiveness in meeting the goals for the preparation of future physicians. We must regularly ask: to what extent do our present educational methods support the learning and caring that must be fostered during professional training—and sustained through some four decades of self-education in the career of each physician? At Harvard and, indeed, across the country, with support and direction from such organizations as the Association of American Medical Colleges, the Institute of Medicine and the Macy Foundation, this question is being taken up with renewed interest.

Faculty and student members of Harvard Medical School

have been considering again some of the fundamental questions in medical education, and have been actively engaged in planning a new curriculum for students in the Oliver Wendell Holmes Society. Our goals for the new society are threefold. We seek to produce:

—Physicians equipped with a perspective on biological systems that is of sufficient breadth, depth and flexibility to enable them to cope with a complex and rapidly changing world.

—Physicians who are committed to the ongoing exercise of their abilities to learn in medicine; who approach knowledge differently, having developed skills that enable them to acquire and use knowledge well; who are comfortable with and can make effective use of information managing technologies in learning and practicing medicine.

—Physicians who are sensitive to the kinds of caring that underlie the learning and practice of medicine; who are in touch with the world of the patient, and with the personal side of doctoring; who are concerned about and responsive to the moral and ethical issues that arise from the applications of new medical knowledge.

The new curriculum will be conceived as a continuum, interweaving clinical science with the arts and sciences basic to medicine. Essential knowledge will be learned in concert with attitudes and skills, and will, whenever possible, be captured in the form of problems or cases that will be worked by faculty and students together. We recognize that both unity and diversity of goals characterize medical education. A general medical education should not be a lockstep march through a regimen of required exercises, but should offer both a common itinerary and opportunity for in-depth, individual exploration.

Education in medicine, whose knowledge base is never stable, should emphasize methods as much as content. Students should be given fewer "answers" and more tools—tools for self teaching; for synthesizing, framing and revising knowledge; for keeping pace with a rapidly changing profession. They should have the opportunity to practice, from the earliest days of medical school, skills of seeking out information, testing hypotheses, and solving problems. Much of what we want to accomplish has to do with what faculty and students *do* together; we hope to stimulate changes in the attitudes and conceptual frameworks within which faculty teach and students learn. It is our overriding goal to shape an environment of active student learning, for, as Aristotle wrote, "the things we have to learn before we can do them, we learn by doing them."

Summary of the Planning Process

During the past year, Harvard Medical School faculty and students have been developing a plan to achieve the goals for the Oliver Wendell Holmes Society: integration of the basic, clinical and social sciences bearing on medicine; active student learning; and emphasis on the attitudes and skills essential for all physicians. In the pages that follow, the progress of the planning effort to date and the major milestones to be met over the next several years are reported.

In the latter part of 1983, a working structure for developing the New Pathway curriculum was put in place, including a Steering Committee to oversee the planning effort and assume responsibility for policy decisions; eight Curricular Design Groups (CDGs) charged with the development of specific curricular segments; a Curriculum Coordinating Committee comprised of heads of the Curricular Design Groups to establish mechanisms to promote continuity, completeness and integration of the curriculum; and Support Committees to develop resources and personnel in specific areas, such as Educational Methods, Information Technology, Faculty Development and Program Evaluation.

During a Planning Retreat held in September 1983, a list of guiding rules, principles and definitions was developed, and the areas of responsibility for each Curricular Design Group identified, as follows:

1. The Patient: Needs and Desires for Services from Physicians
2. The Doctor: Roles and Skills in Caring for the Human Body
3. Human Biology I: Structure and Function of the Human Body

4. Human Biology II: Identity and Defense
5. Human Biology III: Information Processing and Behavior
6. Human Biology IV: Metabolism of Matter and Energy
7. Human Biology V: Human Life Cycle
8. Experiences in Patient Care

The charge to the design groups was "To create a curriculum for the general medical education of students in the Oliver Wendell Holmes Society. The curriculum design should serve to integrate active student learning of the knowledge, attitudes, and skills in the basic sciences, social sciences, and clinical sciences that are essential for all physicians." Initially, so as not to hamper creativity, each Curricular Design Group worked without instruction concerning allotment of time or responsibility for implementation. The CDGs were urged to consider both the systematic exposition of knowledge within their area of responsibility, and the educational process that will help students develop the attitudes and skills that all physicians should share. They were asked to make recommendations for the integration of basic and clinical science and the sequencing of content in their area of responsibility, to specify prerequisites, and to identify parallel or intersectional relationships with other Curriculum Design Groups.

The eight Curriculum Design Groups met regularly during the winter months, and written reports on their activities were submitted to the Steering Committee in early March. The reports summarize each group's recommendations for educational methods, curriculum topics and content sequencing in its area. These reports were reviewed by the Steering Committee at a day-long planning session on March 10, and a preliminary draft of an overall Oliver Wendell Holmes curriculum was formulated. Two weeks later, the Steering Committee and Design Group Chairmen met to revise and refine this plan.

The Support Committees established to facilitate development of the Oliver Wendell Holmes curriculum have also made substantial contributions to the planning process. These include: the development of a model for Program Evaluation; a detailed sourcebook on Educational Methods; initial goals and strategies for Faculty Development; and a plan for systematic extension of

Information Technology to all phases of the program.

This report describes the overall goals and general guidelines of the Oliver Wendell Holmes Society; an outline of the four-year course of study; proposed educational methods; and reports from the Support Committees on Faculty Development and Information Technology. We emphasize the preliminary nature of the proposed new curriculum. It is our hope that the recommendations contained in this report will stimulate a productive exchange of ideas, and we invite your comments and suggestions.

Overall Goals

A. Attitudes and Professional Characteristics

The professional characteristics of outstanding physicians are listed below as amplifications of the essential qualities of competence: compassion, sensitivity, honesty, integrity, dependability, and responsibility. These affective goals seek to express the ideals toward which students and faculty jointly strive in their determination to become both skilled and compassionate healers. Thus, we expect each student to work toward the following:

1. Attitudes toward patients and colleagues:

   a. Primacy of the physician's responsibility to and concern for the welfare of the patient.

   b. Respect for the privacy and rights of patients.

   c. Sensitivity to the feelings of patients, colleagues and co-workers.

   d. Capacity to be with the sick and suffering and to remain open to their needs.

   e. Determination and energy to do the work necessary to help patients.

   f. Capacity to inspire and fulfill the trust of patients and family intimates.

   g. Respect for, and appreciation of, the contributions of all others participating in patient care.

2. Attitudes toward society at large:

   a. Concern for the health needs of all members of society.

   b. Appreciation of the relation (and tension) between the physician's responsibility to her/his own patient and the physician's responsibility to the needs of society.

3. Attitudes toward learning:
a. Intellectual curiosity.
b. Commitment to continued learning.
c. Desire for intellectual rigor.
d. Awareness of the extent of ignorance (i.e., lack of knowledge shared by all physicians).
e. Ability to reexamine one's premises and assumptions.
f. Commitment to teaching.
4. Attitudes toward one's self:
a. Ability to cope with stress, uncertainty and disaster.
b. Recognition of one's own limitations and willingness to ask for help.
c. Willingness to act in the absence of certitude.
d. Recognition of how financial aspects of practice affect self, patients and society.
e. Recognition of the impact of power on self, patients and co-workers.
f. Ability to set limits and to balance demands of personal and professional life.
g. Awareness of how one's feelings, values and background affect interactions with patients, family, colleagues and co-workers.

B. Skills
1. Acquiring information from and about patients:
a. Interviewing and listening attentively.
b. Observing accurately and incisively.
c. Selecting appropriate technology to obtain clinical information (recognizing its pitfalls and margin of error).
d. Being aware of the cost-benefit relations in using diagnostic technology.
2. Obtaining, retrieving and storing information:
a. In the mind.
b. In print (libraries).
c. In machines (computers).
d. From colleagues.
3. Working effectively with one's peers and the health care system.
4. Communicating effectively with patients, families and colleagues.
5. Performing basic diagnostic and therapeutic procedures.

6. Problem solving:

a. Collecting, organizing and analyzing information in relation to a specific problem (e.g., asking significant questions, setting priorities and planning effectively).

b. Seeing the inter-relatedness of problems.

c. Reasoning through problems and reaching probabilistic judgments.

d. Assessing the validity of information, including research articles.

7. Self awareness.

C. Knowledge

We expect each student to acquire:

1. An understanding of the patient as a living being:

To understand the central physical, chemical and biological principles and mechanisms that underlie human health and disease, including awareness of the natural history and manifestations of disease.

2. An understanding of the patient as an individual and as a social being:

a. To understand the emotional, psychological and cultural underpinnings of human behavior, including the interweaving of mind and body in illness and health, and the dynamics of maturation and aging.

b. To understand the social and cultural determinants of health and disease.

c. To know the financial and organizational aspects of health care.

3. An understanding of the principles of prevention and of therapeutic strategies:

a. To understand the various factors which contribute to the prevention of illness.

b. To know principles of interactions between the human body and substances that may be therapeutic and/or toxic.

c. To understand common therapeutic strategies such as drug therapy, surgery, psychotherapy and radiotherapy.

4. An understanding of the statistical and probabilistic aspects of human biology and clinical medicine.

5. An understanding of the complex texture of knowledge and the importance of detail, achieved in part through in-depth study of a particular subject.

General Guidelines

A. Schedule

1. The school year will consist of 40 working weeks, and will begin in September.

2. The work week will consist of 55 to 60 hours.

3. Sixty percent of the student's effort will be devoted to experiences shared by all New Pathway students. The remaining 40% will be reserved for the in-depth pursuit of subjects of special interest to the individual student, guided by his or her preceptor.

4. For the shared 60%, the total number of classroom hours per week will not exceed 15 hours, including:

	Hours per week
Lectures	*5*
1 Lecture a day	
5 Lectures per faculty member	
Problem-Based Tutorials, Labs, etc.	*10*
Unscheduled individual preparation	
and study time for the 60%:	*15-20*

5. For the individual 40%, the total number of classroom hours per week will not exceed 10 hours.

B. Curriculum Content and Design

1. The Fellows of the Oliver Wendell Holmes Society will, as a faculty body, be responsible for setting the learning objectives for the New Pathway, and for designing a plan to achieve the objectives.

2. Students of the Oliver Wendell Holmes Society will be responsible for setting their own individual learning objectives, and for meeting the goals and objectives of the Society.

3. The general medical education of students in the New Pathway is conceived as a continuum, marked by:

—Longitudinal and sequenced educational experiences.

—Integration of content in a way that supports progressive reinforcement of learning.

—Ongoing relationships among faculty and students.

—Ongoing assessment of the student's professional development.

4. The Fellows of the Oliver Wendell Holmes Society will be responsible for identifying the knowledge, skills and attitudes essential to general medical education, and for designing a curriculum that enables students to master these essentials.

5. The clinical and basic sciences, humanities and social sciences bearing on medicine will be integrated throughout the curriculum.

6. Clinical and basic science faculty of the Oliver Wendell Holmes Society will jointly plan and implement the course of study for the duration of the program. Holmes Society students will be invited to participate in program planning at all phases.

7. The New Pathway will address the full span of general medical education, and will provide an educational experience that is complete and inclusive.

C. Educational Methods

1. Pedagogical methods will follow from and be compatible with the stated learning objectives.

2. The Oliver Wendell Holmes Society will be based on a shared partnership among all participating students and faculty. Educational methods will be designed to reinforce cooperative learning and collaboration.

3. There will be an emphasis on learning rather than teaching; educational methods will promote active learning, questioning, problem-solving, and critical thinking. Experiential and problem-based learning will be primary methods of pedagogy.

4. Independent learning, self assessment, and the use of computers as educational tools will be emphasized.

5. The development of information gathering, management and analysis skills will be emphasized.

6. A thesis describing an independent project will be required.

D. Evaluation

1. Ongoing diagnostic feedback on student performance will be provided through faculty, self, and peer assessment.

2. Mastery of educational objectives will be ascertained through formal evaluation procedures.

3. The curriculum will be evaluated for its effectiveness and changed when necessary, as will the overall goals and objectives of the society.

The Curriculum

The curriculum design is framed in three levels:

Level I outlines in broad strokes a four-year sequence of curriculum topics and educational experiences.

Level II lists the lecture, tutorial and conference topics and educational materials.

Level III details the work schedule for any given week.

The Oliver Wendell Holmes Curriculum will reflect an attempt at integration on several levels:

a. Across traditional basic science disciplines.
b. Across traditional clinical disciplines.
c. Between basic and clinical science.
d. With the medical humanities and social sciences.

The relative amounts of time devoted to basic and clinical science are not expected to differ significantly from their current distribution; rather, the difference will relate to their placement and sequence in the curriculum. Guided by the assumption that learning is enhanced in a pedagogical experience combining both basic and clinical science, we propose a pattern which interweaves the two.

A. Human Biology Sequence

This sequence consists of themes derived from the contributions of the five Human Biology Design Groups. The preliminary plan suggests ways in which material from each design area might be interwoven, and extends basic science learning over the entire four years. While we have sought ongoing longitudinal integration, elements of block design have been preserved, since some material, such as that related to structure and function, may be best learned in a concentrated format, while other material is more suited to longitudinal integration.

The five Human Biology areas—Structure and Function, Metabolism of Matter and Energy, Identify and Defense, Information Processing and Behavior and Human Life Cycle—represent a mixed conceptual framework. By this organization we intend to address both the properties of living systems in their normal and pathologically altered forms, and the overall integration of these systems from the perspective of normal and abnormal development during the various stages of the life cycle.

During the first two years, students' learning will be largely shaped by their studies in Human Biology. Concurrent clinical experiences, issues pertaining to the doctor-patient relationship, and topics in the social sciences and humanties will be organized as directly relevant amplifications of the particular Human Biology topics under investigation. Normal and abnormal physiology and structure will be integrated throughout the course of study.

In years three and four, when hospital-based experiences will form the dominant educational mode, continuing exposure to basic science and opportunity for in-depth study of the pathophysiological mechanisms of disease will be provided in several ways:

1. Weekly tutorials during the clinical rotations, in which basic science issues raised by the patients seen may be systematically explored.

2. Three separate month-long periods devoted to pathophysiology, and analysis of basic science problems raised by cases seen in previous clerkships.

3. Advanced study in basic science and pathophysiology during a three-month New Pathway Subinternship in year four.

B. Experiences in Patient Care

Patient care experiences will form an integral part of the New Pathway curriculum from the first weeks on. In close integration with basic science learning, a logical and gradual patient care sequence will be developed, beginning with the essential rudiments and building on these in systematic fashion. The student's first experiences will be in the role of a lay person engaged in lay language with a patient. There will be no ICM course in the new curriculum. Instead, there will be a longitudinal experience, beginning in the first week of medical school and lasting into the second year, that would have as its goal the rigorous teaching and evaluation of examination and interviewing skills. Step-wise progression through the fundamentals of history-taking, differential diagnosis and, eventually, the full work-up and assessment of patients will be accomplished through Clinical Skills Sessions. There will be use of videotapes, surrogate patients and a variety of clinical settings; this will be supplemented by an ongoing relationship with a practicing physician faculty member in his or her office. Longitudinal patient experiences, correlated with the Human Biology sequence on the Life Cycle, and continuing over the four-years of study, will permit students to consider: what is the life history of the patient, and what happens to the patient after medical treatment?

In the third and fourth years, newly-designed Oliver Wendell Holmes Society clerkship-basic science sequences and a subinternship experience will call for the participation of Holmes Society faculty from the Human Biology, Doctor and Patient design areas. These will form a series of integrated experiences, combining responsibility for the clinical care of patients with continuing exposure to the basic science and humanistic issues raised by the patients seen.

C. Patient/Doctor Topics

We plan to provide students with a wide contextual understanding of the patient's experience, and of the structural, social, political and economic aspects of physician practice. The optimal inclusion of the many disciplines required to illustrate these principles will occur through integration with the other Curriculum Design Groups at each step of the program. Therefore, throughout the four years, there will be weekly 2-3 hour sessions* on topics related to the patient-doctor relationship, in the belief that the significance of this material will be revealed more clearly if it is part of the ongoing educational experience, and if students need to consider these issues repeatedly. A variety of educational formats will be used: lectures, tutorials, clinical experiences, films, videotapes, field trips, home visits, guided readings, etc.

We propose to build on the skills and knowledge which students bring to the initiation of their medical studies, and, through early exposure to the human dimensions of patient experience and exploration of the student's notions of what it is to be a physician, confirm and validate the attitudes which attract students to medicine. The new curriculum will be responsive to the critical experiences encountered uniquely by each student in

---

* Or, an equivalent amount of time may be allocated differently when indicated by the subject matter.

the process of becoming a physician—experiences such as the examination of the first patient; the first exposure to a cadaver; the first experience of having a patient die while under one's care. Self learning, introspection and small group discussion will be emphasized, and all students will participate in a support group with a trained leader. The support group will act as a reference point for the establishment of group cohesiveness, and for self-scrutiny.

The Curricular Design Group on the Doctor saw that its general charge was to influence the curriculum in two important ways: to produce physicians who are more sensitive and who possess better communication skills; and to produce physicians who are more rigorous in their thought processes and in their performances of doctoring skills. We have by no means reached consensus as to how best to accomplish the dual, and seemingly contradictory, goals of increased sensitivity and increased rigor. However, it is clear that strategies for attaining these goals must be fundamental to the ongoing educational experience.

From the beginning of the first year, students will begin to learn "doctoring" and reasoning skills, will reflect on the implications of physician roles and skills, and will develop skills of doctoring over the course of the program. Interviewing and physical diagnosis skills will be learned during the sequenced Experiences in Patient Care that are described above. Opportunities to develop skills of self-learning, information management and clinical reasoning will be woven throughout the curriculum at all phases. Principles of biostatistics, epidemiology and cost effectiveness analysis will be introduced and developed through sequenced clinical cases. And time will be devoted to exploration of the developing physician's attitudes toward self, toward colleagues and family, and toward the patients he or she will eventually serve, as well as to an examination of physician roles, historical changes in these roles, and role changes during the life cycle of the individual physician.

Encompassed under the rubric of "Patient/Doctor" is material now taught within the areas of Social Medicine, Social Psychology, Medical Ethics and Philosophy, History of Science and Medicine, Medical Sociology, Medical Anthropology, Health Policy, Epidemiology and Behavioral Medicine. While the precise sequencing of this subject matter remains to be worked out, topics will be closely integrated with the human biology and clinical experience sequences.

Educational Methods

Any effective educational program must successfully integrate educational goals with educational process and methods. The educational methods utilized in the New Pathway will emphasize "active learning"—the engagement of the student in the formulation of questions, problems, directions and responses needed to define his or her learning. The following outlines the proposed general educational methods to be utilized in the New Pathway Program.

A. Statement of Goals

Students will receive detailed statements of educational goals and objectives, both at the onset of their course of study and before each new unit of the curriculum.

Clarification of educational goals initiates a critical cycle which begins with objectives, moves to course design and to the methods by which the faculty will teach and the students will learn, and ends with evaluation of the individual student and of the overall curriculum. This feedback loop will be an integral part of the teaching methodology.

B. Tutorials

Problem-based tutorials will comprise a major segment of the teaching activities for Holmes Society faculty and students. These tutorials will consist of between five and eight students working with a preceptor, who will use a problem to explore basic science, clinical and psychosocial issues. Problems will be selected to elucidate fundamental concepts and principles. The preceptors will be guided by general educational objectives and, within these boundaries, will encourage students to determine what questions to ask, which research strategies to pursue, and how to acquire necessary information. The tutorials will meet for several hours, and students will then be responsible for gathering information and consulting with resource faculty. This self-directed learning experience will be an important feature of the new curriculum.

C. Clinical Biological Conferences (CBC)

Large group conferences that may involve more than one New Pathway class (25 to 80 students each) will be used particularly to teach clinical problem-solving and decision-making. Case histories will be selected to emphasize psychological, social, economic, ethical, legal and personal issues as well as biologic and pathophysiologic correlation; these case discussions will serve to enhance interdisciplinary integration and the acquisition of knowledge. The considerable experience in this methodology that has been gained at Harvard Business School will be drawn upon in developing these conferences.

D. Longitudinal Preceptor Relationship

Each pair of Holmes Society students will work closely with a basic science tutor and a clinical preceptor during the entire four-year course of study. Preceptors will advise and guide the students, and may also participate as teaching faculty in some portion of the curriculum.

E. Clinical Skills Sessions

These sessions will be conducted primarily in tutorials, with larger sessions used when teaching methods can be effectively applied. Learning methods will include the use of audiovisual materials, videodisks, computers, student self-examination and programmed patients. The educational objectives of these sessions will include:

—Interviewing; communication skills
—Physical examination
—Physician roles, attitudes, socialization
—Clinical reasoning; principles of scientific inference; quantitative methods
—Learning skills; use of computer, library, reading the literature

Clinical skills sessions will be led by a clinician with background in the human biology area under study, and will draw upon the expertise of resource faculty in the basic and clinical sciences as needed.

F. Experiences in Patient Care

Students will have contact with patients from the beginning of their first year. Starting with patient interviews, and progressing step-wise through the fundamentals of history-taking and physical examinations, the students will see patients in a variety of settings, including ambulatory, in-patient, nursing home and chronic care facilities, home visits and in social service settings. Clinical experiences will occur in groups of two, with a single master clinician as preceptor, preferably throughout the entire medical school experience. Clinical problems will be linked to curriculum content areas, and will include opportunity to:

—follow a pregnant woman through delivery and neonatal period
—have a continuity experience in ambulatory care
—interview physicians at all levels of experience and from both basic science and clinical medicine
—follow a patient with a terminal illness
—see patients in a hospital setting without ongoing clinical responsibility, allowing students to focus on the integration of basic science, pathophysiology, behavioral medicine, and clinical medicine
—explore different clinical settings to assist in career choice
—assume responsibility, under supervision, for the clinical care of patients.

G. Curriculum Content Guide (CCG):
The Curriculum Content Guide will be a workbook designed to give support and direction to the self-directed learning experiences of Holmes Society students. With written materials and relevant references, the Curriculum Content Guide will serve as a resource for the student seeking to fill in gaps in his or her knowledge. It will systematically outline, for each component of the curriculum, detailed knowledge objectives, study questions, educational resources, and readings for further study. It may serve as a first reference source for Holmes Society students, prior to other educational activities. The Curriculum Content Guide will be electronically stored and updated yearly.

H. Lectures
A series of lectures, limited to no more than one per day, will be given throughout each medical school year. These lectures will comprise a "signature" series for outstanding HMS faculty lecturers, with a minimum of five lectures given by each speaker. They are intended to illuminate, rather than to cover completely,

the content which will be systematically outlined in the Curriculum Content Guide.

I. Computer-Based Learning

Because of the importance of computers in the learning plan and their role in the future process of delivering health care, we highlight their use as a learning methodology. Each student in the Holmes Society and each core faculty member will be given a microcomputer, which will be networked to a larger, central minicomputer. The computer will be utilized for word processing, data base development and management, computer-assisted learning, and data base and literature access. Electronic mail will enhance and ease communication among faculty and students. Students will learn to use the computer to facilitate their management of clinical data, developing an electronic "notebook" personalized to their clinical needs. Evaluation methods will increasingly draw upon the interactive capability of the computer.

J. Elective or Individual Study Time

Approximately 40% of the New Pathway curriculum will be reserved for individual experiences designed to meet the special educational goals of each student, under the guidance of a Holmes Society advisor-preceptor. Elective experiences may be individual (as in research, work study projects, or home study courses) or group activities. The latter could include elective course work at HMS, MIT or Harvard University, or courses specifically designed to meet the needs of Holmes Society students. Elective experiences might include specially directed learning experiences in groups of 4 to 6, or field work with an international, domestic, rural or urban health project.

K. Evaluation of Students

Student evaluation policies inevitably influence both what and how students learn. Students in the Oliver Wendell Holmes Society will participate in ongoing evaluation and feedback, based on the stated educational goals and objectives of the program. Both formative and summative methods of evaluation will be used to assess the student's medical knowledge, clinical reasoning and problem-solving skills.

On matriculation, a statement of goals and learning objectives will be made available to each student. A faculty advisory network will closely monitor progress, and will provide regular feedback to the student and to the student's preceptor. The primary evaluation of students in the New Pathway will focus on a statistically valid sampling of the knowledge, skills and attitudes required of the graduating physician. Most evaluation will be "open book"—personal, frequent and informal. Ongoing feedback and overall appraisal of the student's interpersonal, attitudinal and skill development over the four years of the program will be provided by the student's preceptor, in a format that can be used as a basis for later reference letters.

Students will be evaluated for their general knowledge, problem-solving and clinical reasoning abilities in each unit of the curriculum. A list of "guiding questions," with accompanying references and supporting materials will direct the student to the key principles, concepts and learning issues in that unit. Students will be evaluated on their responses to a selected set of these "guiding questions." In addition, student mastery of essential knowledge will be appraised by means of self-directed testing in each curriculum unit, in a format similar to the self-study guide of the American College of Physicians' MKSAP.

To assess clinical competency, the student will be tested at several points using programmed patients, which allow valid cross-student and intra-student comparisons over time. Standardized patients provide a reliable means of testing for the acquisition of skills, attitudes and knowledge in the clinical arena. A regional resource for training patient evaluators is being developed at University of Massachusetts, Worcestor, under the direction of Dr. Paula Stillman.

Overall evaluation of the student will be competency-based. To accomplish this, students will be required to respond satisfactorily to a randomly selected and statistically significant sample of the total set of guiding questions. The student will come to the Holmes Society Teaching Center at any time, and will be expected to respond within a generous but defined period of time. Graduation will require successful completion of this hurdle.

L. National Board Examinations:

New Pathway and other HMS students will operate under the same policy with regard to the NBME requirement for graduation. We propose that a special HMS task force re-examine the board examinations for their appropriateness as an evaluation instrument for either the New Pathway or the existing curriculum.

Faculty Development

Teaching activities in the Oliver Wendell Holmes Society will be somewhat different from the ones currently undertaken by faculty. There will be fewer lectures, and a corresponding increased emphasis on problem-based tutorial discussions, self-paced learning, and close correlation between basic science and clinical materials. In addition, the faculty of the Society will have a more sustained interaction with students, and some will serve as advisors and tutors to individual students.

A part of the planning includes the development of a Harvard/Danforth Center for the Improvement of Teaching. Using videotape recordings and expert consultation, individual faculty will be offered assistance in improving lecturing, tutorial skills and case-method teaching.

Finally, because the teaching responsibilities of involved faculty may be relatively heavier than is true of most faculty, a particular effort is being made to document and evaluate teaching contributions.

Information Technology

Fundamental to any medical school curriculum reform in the 1980s is the requirement to deal with the explosion of knowledge in human biology, the broadening scope of medical science, and the restructuring of the medical care process for the practicing physician. The demand to cope with the exponential increase in facts, information, articles, data, tests, and procedures, together with the new alternatives in diagnostic strategies and in medical management have far outstripped the ability of our medical schools to teach, and of our medical students to learn. We must increase both the efficiency and the effectiveness of medical education and instill the commitment and skills for lifelong self-education.

The New Pathway is strongly persuaded that a valid response to the problem of information overload is to take advantage of computer technology to facilitate student learning. We believe that the easy availability of such technology will enhance the student's ability to master knowledge by decreasing the amount of time and energy required to learn the necessary medical information and master the required problem-solving skills. In the New Pathway each student and each faculty member will have his/her own personal computer workstation connected to a communications network. This system will be used to support the everyday information management needs of the student (word-processing, personal reference files, access to curriculum materials, bibliographic files, etc.), to facilitate the administrative needs of the curriculum (network bulletin boards, electronic mail, and scheduling support), and to provide access to new educational software specifically designed for the new curriculum. We plan to develop and implement computer applications that will enhance retrieval and management of medical information, assist in clinical decision-making, and significantly modify the storage and handling of relevant clinical data.

Important characteristics of the personal workstation and communications network that will be emphasized include the following:

The computer system and the information network will always be available for use by the students and the faculty; emphasis will be placed on using the network communications to facilitate collaborative problem-solving and sharing.

The computer applications will be self-paced, interactive and responsive to the individual student's learning style; a primary focus will be to stimulate and facilitate active learning.

The computer applications will take maximum advantage of graphics, animation and integration of visual images with text.

Applications will be developed to provide a mechanism for systematic assessment (by both the student and the faculty) of student acquisition of the knowledge and skills which are considered fundamental to the New Pathway curriculum.

At the present time, we are actively negotiating with several leading computer manufacturers to provide the computer hardware and software support and funds for application programming development. In addition, we have prepared a "check-out and take-home" computer literacy package which includes a portable computer system. This is being made available to members of the New Pathway planning committees to encourage a better understanding of how information technology applications might be better used in the development of the New Pathway curriculum.

May 1984

How to Begin Reforming the Curriculum

Reed G. Williams, Ph.D.

All medical curricula are based on the assumption that a planned educational intervention into the life experiences of individuals desiring to be physicians will result in higher quality physicians and medical care. There are three primary mechanisms of action through which this end can be achieved: 1) selection of better candidates; 2) creation of a learning environment which provides more learning opportunities, higher quality learning experiences or a better selection of learning experiences; and 3) more effective screening of students to ensure that only well-qualified individuals are ultimately certified to practice medicine. As with therapy, there are also side effects and hazards to be considered in selecting and monitoring the methods used. The challenge to those of us attending the conference on *How to Begin Reforming the Medical Curriculum* is to suggest altered approaches to educational intervention in such a way that the desired effects are achieved and the associated hazards and side effects are decreased.

In this paper I will disregard issues related to selection of medical school applicants. I have little to contribute on this subject and am convinced that most individuals who apply to medical school have the potential to be competent, even excellent physicians given proper instruction. Rather, I will provide thought on the nature of instructional environments which are capable of improving on the learning which an individual planning to go into medicine would likely achieve alone or through the apprenticeship model of learning common prior to formal medical education. Also I will address one of the practical problems associated with common methods of instruction used in medical education. These problems are the result of the many internal and external political, social and economic constraints faced by medical schools in planning and delivering undergraduate medical education. It is perhaps these constraints more than a lack of understanding of desirable teaching/learning conditions which result in a compromised instructional approach with a number of hazards and adverse side effects. The perspectives articulated in *Emerging Perspectives on the General Professional Education of the Physician* show that many faculty are well aware of problems with current teaching approaches used in medical education. The document also clearly suggests more appropriate approaches to teaching and learning in abstract form. The diagnosis has been made and general suggestions for improvement have been provided. The real challenge is to develop/select and orchestrate use of specific teaching/learning approaches which are consistent with learning theory and research, pointed toward fostering achievement of the desired competencies demonstrated by expert physicians, and practical given the constraints faced by medical schools and their faculties. In some cases our efforts should also be directed toward modifying existing constraints in the interest of improving medical school instruction.

Tasks of the Expert Physician

A number of excellent studies have been conducted over the years to describe the component competencies required of expert physicians (e.g. American Institutes for Research, *The Definition of Clinical Competence in Medicine;* American Board of Pediatrics, *Foundations for Evaluating the Competency of Pediatricians;* Elstein, Shulman and Sprafka, *Medical Problem Solving: An Analysis of Clinical Reasoning).** Such studies have varied in the level of detail and often have chosen to lump and split competencies differently. However, for present purposes it is sufficient to acknowledge that these competencies fall into

---

* Palo Alto, CA: American Institutes for Research, 1960; Chapel Hill, NC: American Board of Pediatrics, Inc., 1974; Cambridge, MA: Harvard University Press, 1978.

four major classes from a learning task analysis point of view. Physicians in training must learn to: 1) make appropriate discriminations (i.e., note features on an x-ray, hear heart murmurs on auscultation or dullness on percussion), 2) perform technical skills (i.e., percussing a chest or inserting an IV) appropriately, 3) reason effectively about the nature of a patient's problem or the best intervention approach using available facts about the patient and one's own knowledge of human anatomy, physiology, biochemistry, etc., and 4) coordinate knowledge, reasoning abilities, interpersonal and technical skills into a smooth effective performance which achieves a particular goal or set of goals established by the physician for that patient situation. (Hereafter referred to as *executive* or *self-management skills*.) Each of these tasks poses a unique learning challenge and demands somewhat different instructional approaches. However, for present purposes, we will concentrate on those conditions for learning which are common to all four classes of tasks yet are often missing in medical school instruction.

Conditions for Learning

As mentioned earlier, the requirements for mastering the four classes of learning tasks differ somewhat. However, these differences are minor in comparison to the conditions for learning shared by the four. In this section I will discuss those conditions which are most important contributors to effective learning and discuss the implications for undergraduate medical education.

Students have to do the learning. Learning is an active individual process regardless of the nature of the learning task. Students must have multiple opportunities to practice if they are going to learn to detect nicking of capillaries in the retina or hear splitting of first and second heart sounds. They will learn to detect differences in muscle strength through practice as well. In order to reorganize knowledge effectively so that it is retrieved at appropriate times in working with patients, students must learn the content of medicine in the context of solving patient problems. Likewise they should have multiple opportunities to apply this knowledge to later problems. Finally, students can only learn to coordinate their use of knowledge, reasoning, interpersonal and technical skills into a smooth effective performance (i.e., think on their feet) through multiple opportunities to practice.

Too much of current medical school instruction appears to be based on the assumption that listening to a well-organized faculty presentation of basic science information will result in well-organized, easily recallable knowledge in the memory of students or that a presentation on ascertaining the relative strength of a patient's left and right arms will easily translate into the ability to perform this task effectively. This same logic seems to pervade most conventional medical education practices whether the task is to help students learn to relate effectively to patients, to interpret x-rays or whatever. While responsible people disagree on the utility of instructor-organized presentations as an important part of instruction and on the placement of practice in the instructional sequence, all psychologists would agree that the ultimate organizing of knowledge and acquiring of performance capability must be accomplished by the learner and requires a great deal of practice. Further, experts would agree that reserving practice activities for the last two years of medical school is not effective learning strategy. Students should start using knowledge to solve medical problems at the same time they acquire the knowledge itself. This ensures that the knowledge is stored in memory in usable form and is associated with appropriate retrieval cues. Therefore I would suggest that at least 50% of student time during years one and two of medical school should be directed toward practice of relevant discrimination, technical and interpersonal skills, clinical reasoning activities and use of knowledge in clarifying and resolving patient problems. Early opportunities should be designed and directed so that students are not overwhelmed by difficult problems; problems can be handled in slow motion so that novices have more time to work and think their way through performances when additional practice is necessary or desirable.

Instructional activities that support these types of learning experiences include use of paper simulations to teach reasoning skills and application of knowledge, practical instructors to teach technical skills and examination procedures, practical exercises designed to foster the ability to read and interpret x-ray films, listen to and interpret heart sounds, etc., and standardized/simulated patients to foster the executive/self-management skills used in coordinating all of one's abilities when faced with a live patient with medical problems under normal constraints of time and situation.

Learning requires feedback. Effective learning requires the opportunity to reflect on and plan improvements in one's own behavior. This reflection time is more productively used when one has the benefit of an expert's evaluation and suggestions and the opportunity to observe other individuals perform the same task being learned. The critique of an expert indicates the aspects of one's performance which are weak and those which are strong plus suggestions for improving performance. The opportunity to observe others performing the same task suggests alternate approaches to the same goals as well as provides a basis for comparing one's peformance to that of others with equal and/or more experience.

Typical clerkship experiences provide many opportunities to practice skills. However, it is rare when experts observe the entire performance and are thus in a position to provide the most comprehensive and effective feedback possible. Likewise medical students virtually never have the opportunity to observe experts or other students work up the exact same patient as the student has worked up (i.e., starting with the same amount of information about the patient). Therefore, the opportunity to use others as models in situations where one feels that personal performance should be improved is compromised somewhat. Likewise, many of the more difficult aspects of clinical competence (e.g., clinical reasoning, cue detection) are not apparent under normal circumstances. High quality instruction improves learning through making these aspects of competence apparent to observers and thus the subject of discussion and reflection. The use of standardized/simulated patients provides the opportunity for novices to work up patients previously worked up by other novices and by experts. The novice can thus evaluate his or her own performances for weaknesses and observe the performance of others in looking for ways to improve in those areas of weakness. With standardized patients the novice can work up the same patient again, striving to improve his or her performance through incorporating other approaches to aspects of the work-up.

Evaluation Should Be Diagnostic

Evaluation practices in medical schools tend to mimic those of standardized examination programs such as the SAT, ACT, MCAT, and the NBME as used by residency program directors for selection. However, the purpose of medical education is much more comprehensive than that of these testing programs and this difference calls for a substantially different approach to evaluation. The difference is analogous to the difference between a medical examination for insurance company purposes and one for regular purposes.

Standardized examinations such as the MCAT are designed to help decision makers choose a limited number of individuals from a large pool of candidates. As such, the purpose of the examination is strictly to compare the performance of examinees on a standardized set of tasks. Little or no attempt is made to aid in understanding the specific nature of gaps in knowledge, understanding or performative ability. Likewise, the examining boards have no need or obligation to determine those specific competencies which must be demonstrated before instruction is considered complete and a student will be certified as meeting minimum proficiency requirements (i.e., is considered safe). In a medical education program the collective purpose of faculty is to establish learning goals for students (based on the competencies required of physicians) and to provide instruction which helps move students toward achieving those goals. The instructional process should be iterative and result in students successively approximating the level of competence specified in the learning goals. An evaluation system for educational purposes needs to support this iterative instructional process. The evaluation system must be designed not only to identify those students who have failed to achieve competence but also to help characterize the nature of deficiencies and point toward appropriate remedial strategies. Likewise, the assessment system should be designed with absolute criteria of acceptable performance as decisions about promoting students imply absolute judgments about competence and cannot reasonably be made solely on the basis of comparing a student's performance to that of others.

An appropriate evaluation system for instructional purposes might better be modeled after the diagnostic process used in medicine. Assuming this, the system might appear as follows:

1. Initial tests would occur early and would sample competence by assessing student performance using major indicators of competence. These tests would focus on comprehensive skills and abilities where successful performance automatically implies successful mastery of many other skills and abilities.

2. Scores below the lower limits of competence would be attended to regardless of the performance of other students. Scores out of limits would be disregarded only under unusual circumstances. This approach allows professional judgment to enter into the decision-making process accompanied by the responsibility a professional assumes in making such decisions.

3. In areas where the screening test reveals performance below the lower limits, a series of more costly (perhaps only in terms of time) diagnostic measures would be administered to determine the nature of deficiencies which prevent the individual from demonstrating competence.

4. Results of the diagnostic assessment would suggest specific remedial instruction designed to overcome the problem(s) identified.

5. Testing and remedial instruction cycles would continue until the desired level of performance is achieved or the student leaves school.

It may be desirable to establish a single team of individuals to conduct the in-depth diagnostic assessments for a department or even an entire medical school. This would seem to be especially true for assessment of clinical competence. This task requires a detailed understanding of the components of clinical competence, skill in assessing the individual components and a special interest in the areas of clinical competence and assessment methods.

We have established such a Diagnostic Laboratory for Clinical Performance Problems. Its purpose is to take referrals of individuals identified as having clinical performance problems, as yet undifferentiated, determine the nature of the problem, and to plan an approach to remediation.

This approach to identifying, clarifying and solving clinical performance problems of students has the following advantages:

1. This approach is cost efficient. It avoids implementing a more complex time-consuming evaluation system for all students to improve the ability to differentiate the problems of that small percentage of students who are having problems.

2. The responsibility for diagnosing and managing a student's problems is put into the hands of a small group of faculty who are specially trained for this and who can assure continuity of effort.

3. Such diagnostic efforts require more detailed observation of a student's performance and therefore require special facilities such as examining rooms with adjoining observation rooms, videotape facilities and special diagnostic instruments. Duplication of these resources would be expensive. In addition, duplication of faculty teams would be difficult due to lack of faculty with proper training and interests.

A Matter of Organization

As mentioned earlier, many of the constraints on current medical education practice are practical, organizational ones rather than failures to perceive desirable directions for change. I will address one of these.

While individual faculty, department chairpersons and medical school administrators honestly seek a balance of teaching, research and service activity, there is one feature of the medical school economy which can exert an important influence on faculty division of labor whether intended or not. Specifically, both research and service activities of faculty members have direct monetary consequences for academic departments in medical schools and for the administration. Funded research pays part of a medical school's overhead and covers portions of faculty salaries, thus releasing funds for other uses. Generally some portion of released funds is returned to the departments thus increasing the options and resources available to a department and to the school as well. Clinical service activities have the same direct effect on a department or school's options and resources. There is no such direct benefit received as a result of teaching activities. This difference probably results in skewing of individual faculty and department chairperson decisions and actions toward pursuing and encouraging research and service activities. As mentioned earlier, this is normally not a blatant or perhaps even conscious skewing. It does, however, pose problems for those responsible for teaching programs.

A number of medical schools outside the U.S. (most notably the University of Newcastle at New South Wales) have adopted a financial structure where course directors, or curriculum committees are provided a personnel budget to use in delivering their portion of the curriculum. They in turn contract with department chairpersons for the teaching services of faculty on a yearly basis. In this case, faculty members are more directly accountable for the quality of teaching services in those courses where they have agreed to teach.

There would be more incentive on the part of the faculty and chairperson alike to find a satisfactory combination of assignments for the faculty member. Likewise, the faculty member would be stimulated and reinforced for investing appropriate time and energy in each assignment to ensure success. The yearly renegotiation of teaching assignments would work to sustain attention to quality of teaching activities. This approach should ensure that the perceptions of chairpersons regarding teaching activities are in line with their perceptions regarding research and service since teaching activities of faculty would result in added funds and flexibility for departments.

January 1984

Appendix B:
Reactor Papers

Arnold L. Brown, M.D.

Reformations are not effected by persons who are only casually discontented with the status quo. Reformers are true believers, perhaps not entirely in the Hofferian sense, whose feeling of outrage is matched by an inexhaustible energy and a complete absence of patience for those who defend, or complacently accept, the way things are. In reading the papers written by Abrahamson, Barrows, Erdmann, Neufeld, Williams, and the Smalls, as well as the program destined for the Harvard Medical School, it is clear to me that these represent no casual discontent, nor, to the extent that I know them, is there any lack of energy on their part in the vigor they have exerted in changing the medical curriculum. I do detect, however, a degree of patience for the unenlightened which may explain the presence of "begin" in the title of this symposium. While outrage may be too strong a word to use in an academic setting, there can be no doubt that these authors see little that is good in the present curriculum and feel strongly that the sooner it is changed, in fact recast, the better will our future physicians be.

Two themes appear in these papers, one concerning the process of change, the other the content of the changes. As the dean of what I shall call a mature medical school I shall limit my comments to the change process, the "How to" of the symposium's title. Content, a subject about which I have some fairly strong views, can be left to another time.

First, two opinions. I believe that it is high time that some basic changes should be made in the way we educate medical students. I am also convinced that such changes can be made.

The role of a change agent(s) is never easy and, as Abrahamson has so vividly described, may have dire personal consequences. The first requirement, and to ignore it will very likely lead to those consequences, is to understand the environment. Abrahamson understands this, as do Erdmann, Barrows, and Neufeld, as I read their papers. I shall add some points that are particularly apparent from the dean's office. First, medical schools, as is well-known, are no longer in a growth phase and now must make do with level or, more likely, declining resources. Changes that require funding must compete with programs already in place, entrenched if you will, which leads me to a second characteristic of our environment. Medical school faculties, in common with those of the rest of the university, run their school. This is accomplished through the process of faculty governance, a fact which no dean or change agent can afford to underestimate. Abrahamson deals with this fact forthrightly with his suggestions concerning the involvement of all parties and the need for empathy for those who oppose change. Dean Tosteson must have had this in mind when he determined the size of the group that devised the Oliver Wendell Holmes Society.

It is also appropriate, as Dr. Neufeld has reminded us, to consider the environment outside the medical school. The students who come to us, and our faculties as well, are products of that environment. We must take this into account as we shape our expectations for our students as well as of our faculties in the changes that we have in mind.

The conservative nature of our faculties was mentioned in several of the papers. This is only partially true. When it comes to their research they are alive to the very latest information and concepts. While paradigms may be supported well beyond their usefulness, new methods and new approaches to complex questions are avidly taken up and used. Why then are not the results of research into the educational process treated with equal enthusiasm? I suspect each of you has an answer to this question. At a time when research into medical education has never been greater in terms of the number of papers published there seems to be little if any connection between this body of knowledge and those who could use it.

It is here, perhaps, that we aproach the nubbin of the problem. How do we decide what is the best way to educate a medical student? The answer to this must surely include a definition of the kind of physician that we wish to produce. Such a definition requires, for the benefit of a skeptical faculty, criteria that, at least to some degree, can be measured. Few, if any of us, regard the NBME examinations or any other test to be adequate in this regard. We recognize that we furnish only the initial education and that the next phase is just as important and the one after that is even more so. How, then, do we measure the physician? The answer to that defines our curriculum and makes the process of change, of reformation, obvious.

In the absence of an acceptable measure of the quality of our graduates it is fair for me to express an opinion based on non-systematic observations on wave after wave of medical students and the physicians that they have become. The vast majority are good practitioners, many of them are excellent and only a few should be doing something else. They work hard, remain reasonably current with what is going on in their fields, take good care of their patients, and try their best to fulfill the expectations of those in their care. This is an opinion on my part and a conviction for others. It would be wise to keep this in mind when considering the reform of the curriculum.

Once the dean is energized and the faculty is convinced, not necessarily in that order, that there must be change then, perhaps even before, the content of that change must be explained. Not only must it be explained but is must be justified to a group of people whose professional lives have been spent in the careful scrutiny of the evidence for every assertion that affects them.

The faculty might also agree with Diane Ravitch, who has recently written in a broader context, "Pedagogical practice follows educational philosophy, and it is obvious that we do not yet have a philosophical commitment to education that is sound enough and strong enough to withstand the erratic dictates of fashion."*

April 1984

---

* D. Ravitch, "The Continuing Crisis, Fashions in Education." *American Scholar* 2 (1984):183-193.

William J. Dignam, M.D.

I fully agree with those who have indicated that it will require a major effort to persuade faculties of schools of medicine that major change is necessary. Several of the authors have outlined strategies to be employed and they will certainly be necessary. First, however, it will be necessary to convince faculty members of major problems with graduates who have had present day curricula.

To my mind, and as expressed by several of the authors, the greatest single problem with the graduate physicians is the lack of successful activities to continue their own educations independently. We have not been successful in teaching them to do this during their medical school careers, due in large part to our reliance upon lectures or other exercises in which the students play a very passive role. We make the same error in our attempts to keep practicing physicians well informed. Most postgraduate courses consist of lectures and little is retained by the auditors. Frequently physicians comment that they learn more from having one sick patient and reading vigorously about the condition exemplified than they have learned by attending repeated lectures on the same topic. Yet, we continue to ignore this information and to rely heavily on lectures.

The identification of students who have a genuine thirst for knowledge and who will have the continuing dedication to the welfare of their patients, and therefore continue to seek

132

vigorously for knowledge which will benefit their patients, is an admittedly difficult task. However, it should receive much more emphasis during the admissions process and currently it receives practically none.

An active program of self-education by medical students can only be carried out by their personal participation in laboratories, patient care activities and seminars. Even in these activities students can be quite passive if permitted to do so by unskilled instructors.

I agree with the suggestions of reallocation of time devoted exclusively to basic medical sciences in the curriculum, but I would involve the basic scientists much more heavily in the seminar discussions. This would be good for both the basic scientists and the clinicians. Any decision about time to be allocated exclusively to basic sciences is bound to be somewhat arbitrary. I believe that students do need a period of instruction in the basic sciences and in the techniques of taking medical histories and performing accurate physical examinations before they can benefit appropriately from discussions of clinical problems. I believe that after completing the undergraduate education one month of vacation per year should be sufficient. I would therefore have students start medical school on the first of July following completion of undergraduate education, have 44 months of education, and be prepared to start residency education on the first of July, after a month's vacation.

I would devote 11 months exclusively to the basic medical sciences, to be spent in laboratories and seminars, two months to learning the techniques of patient evaluation, 20 months to seminars concerning clinical problems, and 11 months of assignment to the clinical services. The first 11 months would be conducted by the basic scientists, but no lectures would be permitted. The seminars devoted to clinical problems would be conducted by both basic scientists and clinicians. The biomathematicians would play an important role.

The seminars devoted to clinical problems would be titled by patients' symptoms because that is, after all, the manner in which patients come to our attention. I would structure them in a manner such that the problem would be introduced early in the day, students would disperse to acquire necessary information (possibly receiving some guidance concerning appropriate sources at first) and then the same group would reconvene later in the day to continue the discussion. My own experience would indicate that faculty members will be surprised to recognize how much information is already known to many of the students before the discussion begins.

All of this will require, as a number of authors have indicated, some changes in the attitudes of departments. Departments are essential units for universities. So long as they are not permitted to proliferate to the point where the area of knowledge encompassed is too small they do foster the production of appropriate research to extend the knowledge in that particular area. I believe that the existence of clinical departments does result in better patient care. The particular knowledge extant in the department does permit better education of residents. Departments do not, however, contribute as successfully as they might to the general medical education of undergraduate medical students.

It will be necessary to convince faculty members that they cannot attempt to impart all of the knowledge of a given subject and that that knowledge will quickly be out-of-date anyway. It is quite possible that all of the topics covered in medical school today would not be covered if more time-consuming educational exercises were conducted, but if those exercises were successful in developing students who could and would continue to educate themselves a much more important objective would have been obtained.

I am very much in favor of titling clinically-related seminars by symptoms. I would and do conduct these seminars in the same manner as one evaluates a patient. The patient's background and the possible effect of factors such as emotional factors should be discussed and then consideration given to the possible pathology involved, the manner in which it causes these symptoms, other conditions which may cause the same symptoms, diagnostic measures which may be employed, the possible methods of management, and the results to be expected. A truly critical review of references supplied to substantiate points of view must be a prominent and continuing activity. Here the biomathematicians can play a very important role. This is probably one of the most important features of teaching students to continue their own educations independently in the future. At first it will seem to a basic scientist such as an anatomist or a physiologist that he or she is wasting a lot of time sitting in seminars. The individual contribution is not great but the gains in stimulating relevant teaching during the first year will more than justify the effort. It is true that it will be necessary to devote more time to teaching activities, but at the present time many members of medical school faculties do not spend enough time teaching. To me it seems not at all unreasonable that members of medical school faculties spend the equivalent of 10 hours per week the year around in seminars or teaching laboratories.

The technique of conducting a seminar successfully is not one which comes naturally to some faculty members. It will probably be necessary to teach this technique to faculty members formally. In particular they must learn to elicit the participation of all students present by direct questions if necessary. If this is done there will be no significant problem in evaluating students and no additional tests—objective or otherwise, would be necessary. We have overdone the grading of medical students. One of the primary purposes of such grading is to permit responsible recommendations to directors of residency programs. Excellent performance in medical school does not necessarily portend excellent performance in residency anyway. It is sufficient to identify the top 10% of students and the bottom 10%, leaving all the rest in a "completely satisfactory" group. We do owe our colleagues the identification of the bottom 10%. I believe that dean's letters of recommendation indicate that many, too many, students are "in the middle of the class."

Some very worthwhile strategies for persuading faculties to carry out the necessary changes have been suggested by the participants in this conference. Whereas I recognize the concerns expressed by Dr. Erdmann in his final paragraph and would clearly not want to stimulate a major effort which ultimately proved to be futile, I do believe that a confrontation is necessary and that attempting to solve some of the specific problems, without first convincing the faculties that a major change in orientation is necessary, would not attain the desired objectives.

The suggestions made in the papers of Abrahamson, Barrows, Erdmann, Neufeld, the Smalls, and Williams are all very helpful. They should be carefully considered and implemented wherever possible by the various schools of medicine. I am particularly supportive of the need for faculties to develop a "corporate sense" of responsibility for the general medical education of our students. We must accomplish this if any change is to take place and is to be effective. This has been noted in several of the papers, particularly those by Barrows and Neufeld.

I am concerned about the suggestions regarding remedial instruction made by Williams. I should like to have some information about the ultimate performance of students who have been given remedial instruction. I carry the prejudice that we have been much too reluctant to admit the mistakes of our admissions committees and to dismiss students who do not have appropriate characteristics or do not make appropriate progress.

The new program at Harvard is certainly very interesting and I can agree with much that is contained therein. The statement that graduates will be qualified to enter the second year of the residency program in all clinical specialties is in error. Clearly this is not the case in Obstetrics and Gynecology, and this may apply to some other specialties as well. As presently organized most residency programs in Obstetrics-Gynecology have so much instruction in the necessary skills during the first year of the program that an individual who has not had that instruction could not successfully enter the second year of the program. Therefore, graduates of the new Harvard program would need to start in the first year of the residency. I do not view that as a major problem, but it is possible that the individual students might consider it to be. This is particularly true when several specialties are being urged to extend the length of the residency program in order to provide appropriate education in their increasingly complex specialties.

You asked us to comment upon how reforms could be initiated at our own institutions or those with which we are familiar. I believe that it will be difficult to persuade the faculties of the neccessity for change, but that it would not be difficult to make the necessary changes if the majority of individual faculty members could be convinced of that necessity. As I have suggested earlier, I believe that it will be necessary to emphasize to them that some of the present graduates are not learning to educate themselves independently and that this must be changed. Once faculties have agreed upon that fact I believe that they will understand the necessity for change. I believe that this necessity would best be emphasized by a faculty-wide retreat as noted by Barrows. The plan for implementing necessary changes can be developed by heeding some of the suggestions made in previous publications and in particular the conclusions reached in this present conference.

March 1984

Charles P. Gibbs, M.D.

First, because the title of the conference is *How to Begin Reforming the Medical Curriculum,* and because you indicated in one of your original letters that "our goal is to harvest . . . an agenda that will result in practical solutions for the problems identified in medical education," I have chosen to begin my comments with a description of our plan for review and revision of our curriculum. Following a brief description of the plan, I will relate it to the questions raised in the invited essays.

The review and revision process is to take approximately two and a half years. Because we believed that any curriculum revision should be based upon a thorough knowledge of the existing curriculum, our plan is heavily weighted toward the review process. To guide the Curriculum Committee, we constructed an outline that began by specifying goals of the medical school. We next identified areas of potential weakness in the curriculum (including content, teaching and evaluation). Finally, we listed those concerns suggested by medical educators throughout the country as provided in such documents as the AMA's *Future Directions for Medical Education,* Josiah Macy's *The New Biology and Medical Education* and GPEP's original *Charges to Working Groups.*

Each member of the 16-member Curriculum Committee assumed chairmanship of one or more subcommittees assigned to review each course offered during the four-year medical school curriculum. Committee members attend lectures, seminars and laboratory sessions. On the clinical services they observe the students on ward rounds and in the operating rooms as well as in clinics, some of which require travel to rural areas. Although they cannot attend all lectures and seminars offered by every course, they attend enough functions to develop a solid foundation and "flavor" for what occurs in each offering.

For the basic science courses, the chairman is always a basic scientist. Other members include two clinicians, one additional basic scientist and one medical student. The course director is an ex-officio member and serves as an information source. For the clinical courses, the chairman is a clinician and the committee consists of two basic scientists plus an additional clinician as well as a medical student and the course director. We hope that this committee structure will lead to a better understanding of the clinical portion of the curriculum by our basic scientists and of the basic science portion by our clinicians. Initially, when our basic scientists were asked to serve on committees evaluating clinical courses, they wondered what their roles would be. Several have now indicated that they are enjoying the experience and for the first time realizing what medical students do once the leave the basic sciences. Likewise, several of our clinicians now understand what freshman medical students are taught and what they experience the first two years.

Following the review of each course, the subcommittees meet with the faculty from the course being reviewed, and findings are discussed. Finally, a report is written and submitted to the Curriculum Committee for information and inclusion in the overall curriculum review report. By the time the Springfield conference convenes, we will have completed the review of the first year of basic science courses as well as all of the required clerkships.

Concurrently with the course reviews, the Curriculum Committee is interviewing each department chairman individually to ascertain his particular views, comments and suggestions regarding the curriculum. Following his presentation, an open discussion ensues. In addition to department chairmen, other faculty members particularly interested in medical education as well as private physicians are invited for interview sessions. Also included in these sessions will be guests from other parts of the university, such as the School of Arts and Sciences, the Law School, Dental School and administrative officials. These sessions are well-attended, informative and are held during the noon hour in the Dean's conference room where near-gourmet lunches are provided by the Dean.

Before beginning, the plan was presented to the Dean, Faculty Council and the Executive Committee (chairmen). All endorsed the plan and agreed to participate. Our Dean, Dr. William B. Deal, has been particularly supportive. He has appeared before the Curriculum Committee on two formal occasions to stress his support and provide encouragement. As testimony to that support, he established my position, Assistant Dean for Curriculum, and provides the bulk of my salary. At the end of the entire review process, we will have involved nearly half of our 405 faculty members in the School of Medicine.

Following the review, which should be completed in March of 1985, the Curriculum Committee will make suggestions for change or renovation. By that time, we will have a thorough knowledge of our own curriculum. Also, because literature concerning medical education is frequently distributed to all Curriculum Committee members, the committee will be more knowledgeable about medical education in general. Even at this early stage, it is not unusual for members of the Curriculum Committee to distribute educational material from their own reading experiences to the entire committee. We believe that this rather lengthy process will result in recommendations for change based on facts, knowledge and faculty support.

Response to Invited Essays

I will now comment on the invited essays in light of what we have chosen to do at the University of Florida.

Dr. Abrahamson's cynicism is eloquently and sometimes humorously expressed. I hope he has chosen this mode of expression for its dramatic effect rather than as a representation of his true feelings. Because we have involved a significant number of our faculty and administrators, we hope to avoid many of the pitfalls that he stresses, particularly that of the domino theory. Perhaps the faculty will believe that the "theys" are themselves. Dr. Abrahamson's mood changes considerably during the second half of his essay in which he offers eight very worthwhile suggestions. We believe that our proposed review system address-es most of those suggestions, particularly those dealing with knowing the system, anticipating problems in resistance, obtain-ing administrative support and including all parties.

Dr. Barrows has presented many helpful suggestions in his usual knowledgeable style. He, too, stresses the need for faculty involvement when he says "they (his suggestions) are offered with the belief that a complete and faculty-wide restructuring of educational values and activities is needed to effect any real change."

Dr. Erdmann suggests that this conference might be the place to begin discussing how to implement some of the changes that have been identified by the GPEP project. Certainly, this would seem reasonable. Pertinent to this point, at the recent SGME meeting, results of a survey instituted by Terrence Kuske from the Medical College of Georgia indicated that 36 of 41 schools in the southern region were involved in curricular changes in the years 1980-1983. Moreover, many of those changes were along the direction of those indicated by the facul-ty response portion of the GPEP report, *Emerging Perspectives on the General Professional Education of the Physician.*

Harvard's plan, "A New Pathway to General Medical Edu-cation at Harvard Medical School," is an exciting plan which in-cludes many thoughtful innovations. My major concern, as ex-pressed by Dr. Moy, is whether or not the students will truly be ready to enter into the second year of any chosen residency pro-gram. The logistics of this particular aspect of the plan seem *almost* overwhelming.

Dr. Neufeld provides us, as expected, with a concise sum-mary of the issues and dilemmas. We hope his "corporate sense" among our "community of scholars" will develop during our school's review and revision process. Regarding faculty reward for teaching, our Curriculum Committee recently developed a statement suggesting how faculty teaching efforts can be better documented and thus more evident during review of a faculty person for promotion and tenure. The statement has been ac-cepted by the Faculty Council and Executive Committee.

Dr. Williams suggests that "the assessment system . . . can-not reasonably be made solely on the basis of comparing a student's performance with that of others." Certainly, this is true when we are dealing with medical students. It is sheer folly to grade these students "on a curve." Somehow, we must educate our faculty in this very important aspect of student evaluation.

Dr. Small, a friend and consultant, has collaborated with his two sons to provide another interesting and very stimulating document. Of course, I know Parker's feelings very well and respect them greatly. I am particularly fond of his desires to increase active learning. To do so, he suggests a larger number of appropriate laboratory experiences, small group teaching and self-instructional methods. These are obviously good suggestions, but perhaps the best stimulus to active learning behavior is to modify our evaluation system in a manner that he proposes. Obviously, I do not share his pessimism regarding curricular change.

Before finishing, I want to thank Dr. Moy for informing us about the significance of the academic hood.

Finally, a personal thought. Much of our problems with medical education today would be eliminated if we could only get faculty more involved in medical education and serve as proper role models for students. Faculty need to act like scientists and physicians, and students need to see them doing so and participate with them as they are doing so.

April 1984

Marilyn Heins, M.D.

Instead of specific responses to individual papers, I will briefly list some of my own ideas about curricular reform.

1. Any curricular reform requires a full measure of devotion on the part of the faculty. Today many faculty are on the verge of exhaustion. Picture them stuck full of arrows like St. Sebastian: one barb represents difficulty in obtaining research dollars; another arrow results from efforts at cost containment which alter how physicians practice medicine; still another stems from the new phenomenon of competing for patients. People who grew up in the depression were scarred by this experience; those of us in medical education today grew up in an era of expanding affluence and we, too, are scarred. Some of us may never recover from the shock of today's changes and the implications of these changes. All of this makes it difficult today to identify interested, energetic, concerned faculty who will need to be involved in whatever reform will occur. Those that can be found are often over-committed and over-committeed.

Student stress is often discussed. In Arizona we are also beginning to think about faculty stress and whether we need to consider support systems for the faculty. I believe we are not paying enough attention to the faculty in view of current stresses and think we should try to find ways to help the faculty evolve to their new and inevitable status.

Without question, the primary mission of a medical college

is education. But as dollars drive the system, one cannot provide enlightened education if one cannot pay the light bill. Though dollars are vital, we must also help restore faculty energies so they can fulfill the educational mission of the medical school. On the other side of the coin, some faculty members who prefer teaching to meeting their salary gap, might be energized by curricular reform, as it gives them a chance to do their thing.

2. Although there are many things wrong with American medical education, there are many things right with medical education as well. The medical schools of America do graduate competent and caring physicians. As residents and practitioners they have provided excellent medical care for myself and my family. Two cautionary proverbs: We must avoid throwing the baby out with the bath water. We also should not fix the parts that are not broken. (One wit recently asked why we didn't fix public transportation in America, which didn't work, instead of AT&T, which did.)

3. I totally support the adage that there should be no change without corresponding evaluation. One dimension of evaluation sorely neglected, both in American medicine and American medical education, is patient satisfaction. Let's measure the perception of patients about student performance before and after any major curricular reform. At Arizona we are currently playing with a Patient Satisfaction Scale and are even toying with adding chronically ill patients to the small group experiences we are designing for students. Another area worthy of consideration is peer evaluation, because honest evaluation of each other's performance could be helpful to students.

4. Following the managerial model of "stroke" or "stretch" as the best or, perhaps, only ways to motivate people, I suggest not only local but *national* teaching awards. At Arizona we have an Annual Faculty Teaching Award Day. Students choose the Basic and Clinical Science Educator of the Year as well as the best teaching department in each category. Faculty receive a plaque and a chair to commemorate their honor; each department receives a $5000 allocation to be used as discretionary funds. I propose a National Faculty Teaching Awards Ceremony at the annual AAMC meeting, with nominations coming from the schools and a financial award going to the school which houses the winning faculty.

5. As a revolution may not be desirable or possible, perhaps we can work within the system. Most schools function with a department structure. How about *challenges* to each department in each school to: 1) find ways to remove material from the content they teach as new material is added (curriculum subtraction can obviously cure some of Abrahamson's diseases of the curriculum; it can be applied to any part of the curriculum, especially any part which is in a rapid growth phase); 2) provide small group experiences in addition to lectures; 3) introduce problem-solving exercises; 4) modify examinations to include thinking and problem-solving exercises; 5) change examination scoring to reflect what the student knows, not what he doesn't know; 6) foster self-learning; 7) utilize computer technology, etc. Departments successfully meeting such challenges would be suitably rewarded.

Two relatively simple challenges might significantly change medical education and the practice of medicine. We could reintroduce meaningful laboratory experiences in the basic science years to provide small group interaction, faculty contact, as well as problem solving. Basic science faculty who love and appreciate their science can serve as a model for the students who may even emerge with a sense of curiosity and a desire for inquiry. Second, we could reintroduce a system which ensures that attendings interact with clinical year students at the bedside, not just in the conference room. This provides role modeling of the competent/caring physician in the setting where his competence and care have meaning.

I am looking forward to the privilege of participating in the Macy Conference.

May 1984

Richard H. Moy, M.D.

While there is some appropriate overlap of ideas and recommendations among the seven pieces presented for comment, there is also an impressive diversity of scope, experience and approach which together make a rather complete statement of the problem. Each paper has merit deserving of considerable thought and comment; however, I will restrict myself to those ideas and suggestions which I think are particularly helpful toward a tentative plan for action.

The following is divided into two sections. The first is commentary on the set of thought pieces provided to us and the second is some suggestions related to possible steps toward reform tactics.

Commentaries

A. Stephen Abrahamson

The wisdom of this piece reminds us that there is a full generation of experience represented by heroic martyrs who have hard-won lessons for us to consider. This is a very pragmatic note with which to begin these deliberations.

I was taken with the recommendation of broad departmental and faculty participation so that they will "own" the results. A related suggestion was that proposed changes must reasonably tie-in with institutional value priorities. While not quite so overtly stated, there was a suggestion to key off the pride of the institution and its faculty. A reasonably authoritative voice, internal or external, properly orchestrated, could stimulate action by a proud institution. On the other hand, a fruitful result could be a source of pride and accomplishment and perhaps create an environment with permission for further experimentation. Another note that comes through is that once the reformation has begun, there could be much broader permission for subsequent and ongoing reform.

B. Howard Barrows

Obviously I am very familiar with Howard's thoughts and activities, but as I read his piece two related thoughts came through which I think might be useful to further explore at the Conference. The first would key off the general national discontent, and particularly the General Professional Education of the Physician (GPEP) activities, to enhance an environment in which there is a national "non-permission" for the status quo. Authoritative voices outside of the medical schools, as well as the Association of American Medical Colleges (AAMC), should call for a better quality performance. I would reference specifically the comments of President Bok at Harvard on the occasion of the 200th anniversary of the establishment of that medical school. After many laudatory comments, which were quite appropriate, he did challenge the medical school to do something about its rather traditional curriculum. (I have wondered since hearing his comments whether these were spontaneous by President Bok or might have been suggested to him by Dean Tosteson.)

The related thought is the one which simply must be stated over and over and that is that faculties should clearly be prepared to bring to learning and the curriculum the same scholarship and discipline that they expect of themselves and others at the bedside and the laboratory bench.

C. James Erdmann

I was somewhat troubled by this piece the first time I read it because I know Jim is more creative and probably more positive than originally came across. On second reading, a certain familiarity of the "concerns" suggested what is probably the explanation and that is that Jim is near the epicenter of reaction to the GPEP Study. Some of the deans are staunch products of the last generation of experience in medical education described so well by Stephen Abrahamson. Accordingly, their own careers, as well as their institutions, relate to a different priority system and are not likely to be immediately and intuitively responsive to the curriculum concerns being raised. As they picture going back to their executive committees and powerful chairmen to try to get their attention about needed reforms, I suspect some of them find that they lack the verbiage, leverage, and, in some cases, the commitment to be effective. Accordingly, to follow Abrahamson's metaphor, it is probably better to have the head of John the Baptist than to have to continue to listen to the "voice in the wilderness." Jim Erdmann's battered message is indeed an appropriate warning about the environment but should not dissuade us from trying to come up with practical recommendations for the problems that he presents.

D. Vic Neufeld

Vintage Neufeld, a masterful and practical view of the entire situation along with cogent recommendations presented with an economy of words. While all of his suggestions have merit for discussion, I am particularly taken with the second one relating to the accreditation system. These are not only excellent suggestions which bring in the leverage of the Liaison Committee on Medical Education (LCME), but are quite compatible with their "Essentials." I suspect one thing that will come out rather strongly in our discussions is that the work of individual institutions will be greatly facilitated by more purposeful external expectations.

E. Parker Small

I enjoyed the family dimension here along with the rather fresh restatement of the problems. It was an insight for me that the old laboratory exercises, while often not all that useful in regard to content, did indeed perform the purposes of small group discussions. It is also worth restating the rather sharp tribal demarcation as to how a basic scientist views the "education" of his graduate students as opposed to the "training" of medical students. While the six months basic science curriculum may have to be left to future generations, his call, like Neufeld's, for a different focus of the National Boards may be an entirely practical topic for our discussions. I strongly support his thought that, "It is undoubtedly more important for each medical school to develop a process that will promote and sustain evolution of the instructional program than to institute any specific change." That is an important thought, and we may well do better relating to traditional schools by recommending a process rather than a program.

Parker commends, as did Barrows, a more direct interaction with students in regard to feedback and policy formation. Parker seems to recommend workshops, whereas, if I understand Howard correctly, he was thinking more of students sitting with appropriate structures involved with curriculum policy on an ongoing basis. Finally, in his intriguing suggestion to give the students budgetary funds to reward outstanding teachers, I could not help but think that this would take us back to medieval times when scholars wandered the streets of Paris in caps and gowns as a sign of their profession and would lecture students wherever they could be gathered. The students would show their appreciation by dropping coins into the money pouch, which yet today is at the bottom of academic hoods. As the scholar walked the streets and the bottom of his hood would bounce against the back of his legs, the volume of the jingle coinage would continue to display and market his effectiveness as a pedagogue.

F. Reed Williams

Reed recounts four major classes of learning. The same basic dimensions are found in the graduation goals presented both by Vic Neufeld for McMaster and also in the new developing Harvard curriculum. One could not help but be struck at how little of this is amenable to traditional, multiple-choice testing as found on the NBME and FLEX examinations. Reed's recommendations concerning the basic sciences are similar to Parker Small's but somewhat less radical. The diagnostic laboratory for learning problems could potentially be cost-effective not only in terms of dollars (it is estimated to cost between $40-50,000 a year to educate a medical student), but also in human terms concerning the frustration of both faculty and students which occurs from time to time with the risk of making a wrong decision or delaying a correct one.

G. A New Pathway at Harvard Medical School

This is a major and important departure in medical education which has harvested some of the best ideas of the past twenty years with the potential of providing a very influential model. Realizing that the plans are still evolving, I would have the following observations.

I am sure that the faculty at Harvard will be concerned about the "Hawthorne Effect" with this experiment. It is rather unavoidable and I will be interested to see how they control for it. The statement in the second paragraph calls for ongoing reform, as did Parker Small, and I agree with that. It is also compatible with the essentials laid down by the LCME. Previous efforts to try to coordinate the undergraduate college and medical school programs were focused on reducing the time and, accordingly, short-changed the opportunities of a college education. Now, post-GEMENAC*, we can look at better integration of these two major blocks in an educationally sound way which enhances rather than reduces the opportunities for a broad educational experience.

It is certainly notable that Harvard, as recommended by Steve Abrahamson, made a valiant effort to include all constituents in this program at least by the opportunity to comment, if not to be involved with the actual planning. I note and celebrate their acknowledgement for the need to have sophisticated research in regard to establishing valid evaluation mechanisms for the graduation goals they have set out. I think the inclusion of the fifth year is a truly outstanding recommendation and potentially one of the most powerful in terms of national impact.

Again acknowledging that plans are incomplete, I would bring up several things that might retard either the experiment or its model potential. There is no statement as yet of rewards for the faculty committed to this program. Also, Harvard has large faculty resources which might not be available to other institutions. Finally, the identification of outside financial support for

---

* Graduate Medical Education National Advisory Committee

this model is excellent, as long as it is a model, but identification of "on-line" costs should be part of the experiment, since it is not likely that many other schools will get outside funding for starting such programs once they are no longer experimental.

Some Common Areas for Practical Consideration

Among the many recommendations made in these papers, there are some recurring and important themes around which our discussions could focus.

A. Within the Institution

1. Medical schools should clearly admit that they are primarily educational institutions, that this role has an extremely high priority, and that clear goals should be established.

2. The faculty reward system should be modified or clarified (with faculty participation) in such ways that it is reliable for a high quality, scholarly performance related to curriculum design, delivery and evaluation to be successful.

3. Student participation at the policy level should be increased and better regularized.

B. External Factors

1. I think the GPEP findings and recommendations should get the widest possible publicity so that there is no remaining sense of national permission to do nothing.

2. I think that Neufeld's recommendations concerning the LCME are excellent, consistent with the LCME's stated objectives and would certainly add powerful focus.

3. Harvard is accustomed to national attention, but I think that the excitement and experience coming out of the model curriculum should be followed closely, with broad publicity, as an example that even the most traditional of institutions can engage in scholarship related to curriculum without becoming "guilty by association."

4. I think we should consider the role of the university presidents. They certainly cannot ignore a developing national perception that would result from the above three factors and quite possibly, like President Bok, could acknowledge

that their medical schools should get on with the business of being educational institutions. The president, of course, would have to be consistent with his own challenge as he reviews decisions for promotion and tenure.

This external environment could thus provide even the most timid dean with enough external "devils" that he could go back to his executive committee and call upon them to do those things stated in "A" above.

Students

While students are certainly mentioned frequently in the seven papers and in several it is identified that they should be more directly involved with policy development, I think that we may be underestimating something here. The 1960s showed that students are capable of throwing faculty and administrations of institutions of higher education into hopeless disarray with consequences not only of reform but indeed some rather silly remedies that may still take quite a while to undo. While medical students are hopefully more mature and better behaved, there is ample reason to think that in many institutions they are quite angry and cynical. The Swedish sociologist, Gunnarr Myrdal, suggested that the most radicalizing element for a suppressed group is hope. When things are hopeless, they will endure, but when there are clear avenues for hope, they may rise up in an ultimately irrepressible fashion. The GPEP Study and conferences such as this one will state principles and remedies that will appear quite reasonable and attractive to students and will have respectable national and organizational endorsement. For some institutions this force could be more powerful than anything the dean could say and indeed far more embarrassing for the faculty and the chairmen than anything the dean, the president or the board of trustees could say.

With this background, I would then doubly stress the suggestions made about including students in educational policy and reform activities in a very meaningful way. In addition, to follow Steven Abrahamson's reformation metaphor, we must recall that the students are really the only purpose for all this discussion and its ultimate beneficiary; if we have done our selection right they are both intelligent and extremely able. Thus, as a hierarchical system undergoes reformation, there may be a variety of patterns of student participation and responses depending on both opportunities and provocation and the presence or absence of sound leadership. The ramification of these possibilities into all of the various "denominations and sects" could, I am sure, provide the substance for a whole new lecture by Stephen Abrahamson. I would suggest however, that it would be prudent for the AAMC and the American Medical Association (AMA) to be far more purposeful in working with their student organizations concerning curriculum affairs for the next several years.

February 1984

Frederick C. Robbins, M.D.

It is present day conventional wisdom that medical education needs reform and that medical faculties as a rule are resistant to change, a generality that is probably correct. However, we tend to forget that over the past 30 years or so a number of faculties have introduced a variety of changes. The Case Western Reserve University reform was probably the most complete for an established school. But as we all know, some new schools, such as McMaster University, Kansas City, Missouri and Michigan State introduced radically new programs. Many other schools, including Harvard University, (I refer to their earlier efforts, not the present proposal), Duke University, University of Southern California, Stanford University, Ohio State University, University of Washington, Indiana University, University of Illinois, University of North Carolina, and the University of Connecticut, have deviated from the standard educational system to some extent with varying degrees of success. Thus, the situation has not been quite as static as it is often portrayed. However, the changes that generally have been recognized to be desirable, some for three-quarters of a century or more, are not implemented in the majority of schools and it is sad to say, most new schools have adopted programs that are very traditional.

I will make no attempt to comment on each of the discussion papers but from reading the various documents, the following thoughts come to mind.

If change is to take place there must be some perception that there is a need. In spite of the recognition by many people that medical education is not ideal, I doubt that very many faculty are sufficiently concerned about this to give it high priority and this often includes the power structure within the faculty.

It seems to me that the authors of the discussion papers pay less attention to personal incentives of the faculty than they deserve. Statements are made that one must reward teaching. This implies that teaching is not rewarded, and, indeed, in most institutions it is not. However, to change this situation will not be an easy task. The leverage that the dean of the medical school or the administrator of a university has is very limited. The basic science faculty is particularly concerned with research productivity and rightly so because it is this that determines much of their support. In the present competitive world, they cannot maintain themselves without devoting a major amount of their attention to research and to publication. The clinical faculty is equally preoccupied because much of the support for their salaries and departmental activities is generated in private practice or in some mode of rendering service. Thus, the financial incentives are not directed toward teaching, nor is peer approbation oriented in this way. The distinguished investigator or skillful clinician generally receives more acclaim from his peers and the broader society than does the master teacher. Of course, another factor that cannot be ignored and one with which we are all familiar is the difficulty in judging teaching, particularly in quantitative terms. This is a problem that many schools have struggled with, and attempts have been made to provide guidance to promotion committees. However, just as there is a compulsion within faculties to give numerical grades, so is there a tendency to judge faculty performance on the basis of facts that can be quantitated. This is a bit like the drunk who was looking for his hat under the street light, not because that was where he lost it but because that was where he could see. It seems to me that this area is one in which we could invest more effort and even research.

In reviewing the history of American medical education, one is impressed (but not surprised) with how effective the financial carrot can be. The highly successful large-scale effort in biomedical research has been based in the medical schools, and they have responded magnificently. However, the program has been dependent upon the support of the National Institutes of Health, which has provided the necessary resources. In another area, many states and the federal government as well chose to give priority to increasing the number of physicians. This policy was backed up with funds for program and facilities, and the result has been impressive. Now, of course, we are concerned that we have overshot the mark.

External pressure also has been instrumental in increasing the concern within medical schools for primary care and family practice as well as stimulating more emphasis upon the care of the elderly. Examples of the effectiveness of external pressure upon medical school behavior in areas less directly related to the curriculum are the introduction of institutional review boards to monitor human experimentation; more stringent requirements for animal care; and even the creation of that ingenious device, the fifth pathway for American graduates of foreign medical schools. In most of the above instances the external pressure came primarily from government, which backed up its request with resources in order to achieve the stated purpose (the carrot) or made access to certain resources contingent upon compliance (the stick) or sometimes a mixed approach was used. Few institutions could afford not to respond, no matter how much they might wish to. It is hard to argue against the right of society to play a role in determining the kind of health care system it is prepared to support, which includes the behavior of health professionals. However, it seems to me that a valid topic for discussion is how such external forces might be better informed and directed to the benefit of society and yet not impair the capacity of the medical schools to retain independence in establishing their own educational policies and curriculum. One would prefer some mechanism other than the uninhibited political process, but yet it should avoid the appearance or reality or being self-serving.

Other sources of influence external to the faculty are the student body— a resource seldom adequately tapped—accrediting bodies, and external qualifying examinations such as the national or state boards. Again, these can be useful influences, encouraging appropriate change or forces directed to the preservation of the status quo.

In considering how to initiate change one would like to learn from past experience. In reviewing the Case Western Reserve University program, the only one with which I have had personal experience, and which is admittedly unique, the following factors contributed to make change possible:

1. The student body and many faculty were dissatisfied with the very traditional teaching program, dominated by the department chairmen.

2. The new dean was committed to change.

3. A majority of department chairmanships became vacant within a few years, and they were filled with young persons eager to experiment and open to new ideas and cooperation.

4. A foundation grant provided resources to support planning and initial implementation.

5. The faculty structure was changed so that educational matters were the responsibility of a general faculty consisting of most of those engaged in teaching, including some instructors and the clinical appointees. The committee for medical education reported to the general faculty.

6. An administrative structure was created to operate the novel curriculum.

7. Students were incorporated formally in the process of curricular planning and evaluation.

What resulted from this process is well known, and there are various views upon its value, but no one can deny that it was innovative. One of the remarkable features is that the basic principles established 30 years ago still are adhered to and many of the specific programs and administrative structures have endured. It is my view that the structural changes described above are in large part responsible for the durability of the program. Furthermore, it has been possible to adapt to new circumstances, albeit not without many of the same difficulties experienced by all faculties.

It must be admitted that Case Western Reserve University was least successful in reforming the clinical teaching. This was in part due to the constraints of hospital organization, including departments organized according to service needs.

Some of the original programs, such as required student projects and the basic clerkship (a four-month introductory period in either medicine or pediatrics), were given up largely because of the increase in size of the student body, which almost doubled from 1970 to 1976. There is no doubt that increasing the class size presents logistical problems. The proposed Harvard program helps to overcome this for a select portion of the student body but does not deal with the entire problem. We found that the several teaching hospitals developed a healthy degree of competition for the attention of the students, each vying to be the best in teaching. Their motivation was in part pride but also a very practical one because they were attempting to attract the better students to their house staff. This suggests that schools with large student bodies might consider the creation of subgroups of faculty and students who could have some freedom to innovate and compete for student attention.

I am very much afraid that the factors that have been identified as inhibitory to change and innovation are powerful, and many of them are becoming worse rather than better. Furthermore, even in the best of times it is not easy for an institution or profession to reform itself. It is external forces that often precipitate change, and as has been pointed out, this has been the rule in medical education. It is my impression that those charged with setting policy for the benefit of society—this includes various governmental units as well as the governing bodies of universities, medical schools, and hospitals—must exert their influence, and that those of us who are directly involved in medical education must try responsibly to inform their decisions. It is possible that some new mechanism is needed to promote the kind of communication that will lead to more effective decision-making. Like it or not, it is the needs of society that should determine policies, not the welfare of a group of professionals, no matter how worthy.

April 1984

Henry P. Russe, M.D.

As I read the excellent papers sent for comment by the participants in the upcoming Macy/SIU Conference on *How to Begin Reforming the Medical Curriculum,* I was reminded of conversations I had with Dick Moy when he was chosen to become the dean of the new medical school at Southern Illinois University in Springfield. One of Dick's joys at that time was the opportunity to create a medical school embodying the best of the old, yet allow for expression of the best of the new without having an old mold to break or old habits to change.

My own experiences, and those commented upon by the authors of the papers we are reviewing, amply bear out the fact that changing a curriculum can create martyrs, must be done with skill, is often extremely difficult to accomplish and is a process beset by many road blocks and hazards.

Each institution in its analysis of curriculum and design of curricular changes has moved in a direction reflective of specific institutional goals, at the same time following what may turn out to be a common pathway as curriculum evaluation leads to changes throughout the system.

The keen national interest evidenced in several meetings of faculty and students in the general professional education of the physician studies (GPEP) speaks for a growing awareness of the need to review curricular matters at this time. Many of us expect that the activities of GPEP will produce the contemporary counterpart of the Flexner Report which catalyzed so many educational changes in American medicine at the beginning of the 20th century.

Dr. Abrahamson's paper on "The Reformation Movement in Medical Education" is an outstanding essay which probably best captures the spirit of the times as we look to our curricula and consider new shapes and forms balancing the need to impart information and yet imbue students with the spirit of perpetual learning.

I felt that the paper by Jim Erdmann on "Ecology of Curriculum Change" was very discouraging, almost sounding as though we can't get there from here. From personal conversations with Dr. Erdmann, I know that this isn't the message that he intends to impart. I hope that we will hear more of his thoughts at the conference. I agree with his concept that the strategy necessary to produce contemplated change and the analysis of the effects of changes in the curriculum must be carefully prepared and executed.

Reed Williams's paper focuses nicely on the creation of learning environment to provide high quality opportunities for the student. Experience at our medical college and others discussed in the GPEP regional conference almost makes it axiomatic that we abandon the old concept that learning based on lectures is the path of righteousness. The fact is, students attend lectures only when they feel there is something of particular interest to them or something which is going to show up on the examination. At other times, students tend to stay away in large numbers. Dr. Williams's other comments describe some of the processes used in the curriculum at Southern Illinois University, where he and Dr. Barrows are faculty members.

The paper by Dr. Barrows sets out ideas which he has shared with us at Rush Medical College on several occasions in workshops, ideas which in part have formed the basis for our proposal for an alternative curriculum recently approved by the Management Committee and the Board of Trustees. Dr. Barrows emphasizes that a system needs to be developed which focuses on goals and objectives and the accomplishment thereof. He points out to us again that teachers need to be good educators and that the administration of a curriculum is an institutional affair rather than an individual departmental matter.

The points raised by Dr. Neufeld in his paper focused on goals and objectives and the institutional or corporate management of the curricular process, as well as a need for recognition of faculty and the development of appropriate incentives. This is a theme that carries through several of the papers and one which we may wish to spend some time discussing at the conference.

The paper by Dr. Small and sons represented several interesting points of view. I would select the principal message of this paper as being the focus on an appropriate reward system for good teachers.

The emphasis on basic science in this paper was, for me, somewhat confusing, seeming to suggest both that we decrease the amount of time and yet increase the contact between students and faculty going back perhaps to earlier patterns. Perhaps the Smalls will be able to expand upon these thoughts at the conference.

I was particularly interested in the outline of the Oliver Wendell Holmes Society proposal from Harvard Medical School, a new program to be started in 1985. There are many points of congruence in the development of this program and in the comments in papers being reviewed for the conference. There are many points of similarity between this program and the one developed at Rush Medical College.

I should like to present for comment a Proposal for Alternative Curriculum developed at Rush Medical College by Dr. Gerald Gotterer and Dr. Harold Paul. This effort began in 1982 with a two-year phased termination of the off-campus freshman year for 32 of our medical students at Knox College in Galesburg, Illinois and Grinnell College in Grinnell, Iowa. Planning for this alternative curriculum has now been underway for nearly two years; the initial implementation will begin in September of 1984 with a group of eight students, after many labor pains.

I am looking forward to comments of other participants and especially looking forward to the conference.

April 1984

Addendum: Proposal for an Alternative Curriculum for Rush Medical College*

Gerald S. Gotterer, M.D., Ph.D., and Harold A. Paul, M.D., M.P.H.

Historical Perspective

The Flexner Report of 1910 documented and catalyzed changes in medical education which were responsive to the scientific advances being made in the clinics and laboratories of Europe. The changes reflected a commitment to establish medicine and medical practice on a scientific basis. Requirements for entrance to medical schools became more stringent, prerequisites for undergraduate study in biology, chemistry and physics were established, and the medical school curriculum standardized into two years of basic sciences and two years of clinical study. Both instruction and research carried out by medical school faculty emphasized clinical relevance.

The success of directed research in solving specific health related problems during World War II led to a major national commitment to biomedical research with the expectation that illnesses which were major causes of morbidity and mortality could be cured and prevented. This commitment led to startling growth in our understanding of basic biological processes, but at the same time the research interests of many basic science faculty were led away from problems of direct clinical applicability.

---

* This proposal was submitted by Dr. Russe with his reactor paper. Used with permission of the authors.

The medical school curriculum itself has undergone little change since the acceptance of the Flexner reforms. Medical education in the early part of the 20th century was designed to train the general physician. All students went through comparable programs, learned a common vocabulary, and were expected to be competent in all areas.

The first significant post-Flexnerian change was the introduction of elective time into the medical curriculum in 1925 as part of modifications in the program at Yale. Currently, approximately 35% of the time of the clinical curriculum is scheduled for elective study and in many schools the last year of study is entirely elective.

The drift from direct clinical relevance and the increasing specificity and depth of coverage in each discipline occurring during the post-World War II years made process of integrating learned material more difficult for students. In response, the faculty of Western Reserve University in 1952 adopted the second major post-Flexnerian innovation in medical education: interdisciplinary, organ-oriented instruction in the preclinical years. Traditional departmental autonomy in setting instructional objectives was abandoned and instructional units were designed and implemented by interdisciplinary committees. These modifications were tried at other institutions, with success seemingly contingent upon the enthusiasm of the faculty for change and their willingness to compromise the traditional discipline-oriented curriculum.

Most recently more substantial innovation has involved the introduction of independent learning programs and problem-based curricula. Problem-based instruction shifts the central format of instruction from the didactic lecture to the Socratic analysis of clinical problems. This shift reflects an educational reorientation which recognizes not only cognitive content as a major educational objective, but also problem-solving skills and the professional learning process itself.

Problems in Medical Education

Medical student and physician education now takes place in an environment characterized by change, by growth in knowledge of the fundamental medical sciences, by enhanced application of new knowledge to medical practice, and by altering attitudes and expectations by individual patients and society about physicians and health care. In the absence of significant innovation in the educational process, problems have arisen. The discussion below lists some of these which can be observed in the educational programs of almost all medical schools. The list is not meant to be comprehensive, but is provided to highlight educational problems which are addressed by the proposed innovative preclinical program.

1. The current preclinical curriculum is fact-oriented and emphasizes rote memory rather than reasoning and problem-solving.

2. Students have been forced to assess critically the optimum use of their time for study and learning; this frequently leads to poor class attendance, particularly at whole class lectures. This experience has led many to believe that the competence of most medical students is such that they teach themselves the factual content of the curriculum almost without regard to program format.

3. The preclinical teaching program introduces students to the use of current medical literature in only a rudimentary fashion.

4. Increasing costs and limited resources require a critical reassessment of the optimum use of faculty effort in meeting the multiple responsibilities of teaching, patient care, and research.

5. A variety of factors, including conflicting demands on the time of faculty for research and patient care, have led to reduced bedside, patient-oriented teaching.

6. Clinical education, carried out to a large degree in an apprentice format, does not address the clinical reasoning process as a specific learning objective.

7. Professional schools have not taken advantage of the advances occurring in computer technology which will allow students and future practitioners to use computers as memory extenders, consulting-knowledge systems, and decision-making aids.

8. Little attention has been addressed to assuring that students acquire critical attitudes to "given" truths and habits of lifelong learning.

9. Observers with concern about the integrity of the medical profession have focused attention on the effects of the professional education process itself in influencing and molding the attitudes and practices of young physicians-in-training.

Proposal for an Independent Study/Problem-Assisted Preclinical Curriculum for Rush Medical College

An innovative program in Problem-Assisted Learning has been designed to reorganize the curriculum of the first two years in the direction of more independent study. It would have the following features:

1. Thirty-two students will be admitted to the special program for the 1984-85 academic year. Selection will be from a pool of accepted students who will have volunteered to participate in the program and who meet criteria (yet to be determined) for acceptance into the program. Successive cohorts of 32 students will be admitted in subsequent years.

2. Students will be expected to learn the cognitive content of the preclinical curriculum by independent individual and group study, assisted by "resource" faculty and clinical problems as described below.

3. The cognitive content of the curriculum will match that of the traditional preclinical curriculum. The subject matter of the first year of the program will include the vocabulary, definitions, and basic concepts and processes of normal cells, tissues, organs and organ systems and the general principles of pathology, pharmacology, and preventive medicine. In addition, time will be devoted to the organization and handling of information using modern computer technology. The second year will deal with pathology, pathophysiology, and pharmacology and therapeutics, organized according to organ systems.

4. The focus of the study for each subject will be a syllabus prepared by participating faculty. Students will have access to learning examinations and be required to pass a criterion referenced certifying examination in each subject.

5. For each subject covered, a faculty resource person will be identified who will be responsible for assisting in the definition of curricular goals, preparing an appropriate syllabus and examinations, providing supplementary educational support for students, and coordinating in an efficient and cost effective manner additional resources from within the department. Neither the resource person, nor other faculty would be expected to provide formal scheduled lectures. Faculty would be available to suggest additional learning resources and to discuss with students those topics which they might find troublesome or difficult.

6. Students will be organized into groups with eight students in each group. Each group will be staffed by a clinician facilitator who would be a well-qualified general physician. The facilitators will receive special training in the application of the Socratic method to the problem-based approach to teaching and in the group skills necessary for the approach to succeed.

7. The Program will have a director who will: (a) report to the Associate Dean for Medical Student Programs and (b) be responsible for providing necessary guidance and direction so as to assure the success of the program, including, but not limited to: (i) selecting resource faculty and group facilitators in consultation with appropriate department chairpersons; (ii) providing appropriate orientation and training for and coordinating the activities of resource faculty and group facilitators; (iii) assuring that each component of the program is carried out in a manner consistent with overall program objectives; and (iv) providing reports to appropriate faculty committees concerning program development and implementation and student progress.

8. The clinical problem will be the focus of the educational activity undertaken by the group with its facilitator. Clinical problems will be presented in multiple formats, including a written form using the format developed by Barrows (the *"ProBLeM"* book), live or computer simulated patients, or real patients. The cases chosen will be those which will assist in achieving the learning objectives for the subject being studied.

9. The clinical problem will be the primary tool used to train students in the clinical reasoning process. The group will look at an unknown clinical problem, generate hypotheses, look for evidence to support or reject the various hypotheses, identify

pertinent issues for new learning, and then disperse to conduct appropriate inquiry, either individually or in groups. Follow-up sessions will assess progress by continuing the cycle of hypothesis generation and assessment in an enriched way.

10. The group will also provide the format for learning the skills of history taking and physical diagnosis and for formally examining the affective, interpersonal aspects of doctor-patient relationship.

11. The following represents a schedule for a sample week:

	M	T	W	Th	F
9-11 a.m.					
11-Noon	R	R	R	R	R
1-4 p.m.	G			G	
4-5 p.m.					

R: Resource person, office hours
G: Group meetings with facilitators

Unscheduled time will be used for independent group and/or individual study.

12. Student progress will be measured by performance on criterion referenced examinations and in group problem-solving sessions. Plans will be developed to facilitate transfer to the standard preclinical curriculum for students unable to function in the independent study program.

13. Promotion to Year 3 will require passage of: (1) criterion-referenced examinations for each subject unit; (2) measures of the following skills: clinical reasoning, history taking and physical diagnosis, interpersonal skills as applied in the doctor-patient relationships, and (3) NBME-Part I.

14. Since an important aspect of problem-solving and inquiry-based activity involves information processing, the program will incorporate a variety of elements of computer-assisted learning/instruction, as well as text processing and database and file management. The computer activity will be used in a facilitative and ad-

junctive manner, consistent with rational planning, available budget, and the imagination of the involved faculty.

15. The program will be run on an experimental basis for six years and will be developed with appropriate attention to evaluation so that conclusions can be reached about the efficacy of the approach. Options would be retained to expand the size of the program before the end of six years should the program provide early evidence of its success.

Summary

The proposed alternative pre-clinical curriculum shifts the allocation of basic science faculty effort from the preparation and delivery of didactic lectures to the preparation of effective syllabi and serving as expert resources for students. Use of student time shifts from attending lectures to independent study in groups or as individuals. Scheduled student-faculty contact hours are devoted to examining clinical problems which serve as vehicles for assisting independent learning and addressing the currently underemphasized educational goals of clinical reasoning skills and interpersonal skills as applicable in the doctor-patient relationship. Students will have to demonstrate competence in both the traditional cognitive domains, as well as the newly emphasized skills to complete the program successfully.

February 1983

M. Roy Schwarz, M.D.

I. Commentaries

A. Stephen Abrahamson, Ph.D. — "The Reformation Movement in Medical Education: Must There Be Martyrs?"

Of all the things I have read relative to education in the recent past, Dr. Abrahamson's manuscript is a classic. It represents an old pro who has been through many wars, who has licked many wounds, and who is sitting now, looking backwards at what he has learned. This particular manuscript should be mandated reading for every faculty member who considers himself/herself to be a medical educator. I would suggest some additional topics to consider in Dr. Abrahamson's list. Included among these are the following:

1. If you are anticipating making a curricular change, you must define the reasons for the change in a language and currency which the faculty will understand, and hence, support.

2. There must be something in the change for every major unit of the school whether it is something as intangible as pride and honor, or as fundamental as space, FTE or dollars. There must be something in it "for them" if you wish to have their support. There is one institution in this country which is considering the possibility of distributing its state support base on the basis of student contact hours. While there are many positive things in favor of such a

proposal which could be construed as leading to curricular change, the negatives far outweigh the positives in this reviewer's mind. What seems to be happening is that the big departments are forming coalitions to take resources from the smaller departments and to resist any modification of the curriculum which might lead to a change of this nature. 3. The faculty must be challenged if a proposed curricular change is envisioned with arguments such as, "Why can you experiment in sciences and patient care and consider yourself to be on the cutting edge of developments and not be willing to experiment educationally?" In addition, another ploy has been, "Try this experiment for a period, we will build in an evaluation and based on the outcome of that evaluation, we will make modifications." Additionally, the argument of "academic freedom demands that I (we) be allowed to pursue our creative bent; how can you possibly deny me (us) that inalienable academic right?" 4. The lack of reward system for educational efforts and the trappings that go with this reward system including space, FTE, offspring, travel, entertainment funds, and general recognition, make any creative investment in the educational process a very difficult undertaking. "Golden apple" awards don't and won't cut it. We need something new. Should we consider the possibility of separating science-oriented faculty into institutes with different administrative structures leaving behind instructional and patient care faculty in the traditional structure? This might modify the structure such that the organization of the institution to which Professor Abrahamson refers does not become a major impediment to change.

B. Howard S. Barrows, M.D. — "How to Begin Reforming the Curriculum"

I certainly enjoyed reading the paper by Howard S. Barrows concerning the steps that must be undertaken to modify the traditional medical school's curricular program. I am not sure that I share the pessimism that a traditional medical school "cannot make any substantial or lasting changes in its educational programs unless there are fundamental changes in educational administration, faculty knowledge and skills and faculty reward systems." I do agree that the traditional values and rewards have to be replaced with new ones if any significant or lasting change is to occur. What I hear Dr. Barrows describing is a matrix organization, or he is calling for a major administrative change in the structure of medical schools. Additional thoughts are as follows:

1. Do we accept that a failure to continue to adhere to an organ systems curriculum represents a failure or is it an evolutionary step in our understanding? Every medical school which has gone through such a change was modified, in my opinion, for the better regardless of the fate of the curriculum. I would be happy to expand on that opinion based on personal experience, if desirable.

2. Another important question is, "Can the faculty as a whole ever create, adopt, or support something?" This reviewer's answer would be, "no," they must be lead by a small number of people. I am reminded that 17,000 Russians accomplished the Russian Revolution and changed the course of the world. It becomes imperative, therefore, to answer the question, "How do we create similar revolutionaries for medical education if, indeed, we think that a revolution is called for?"

3. I am of the opinion that an administrative change is essential to facilitate lasting educational improvement. Education in a medical school is, in a final sense, a corporate responsibility. It is school-wide in its responsibility and does not rest just in departments. We can never allow the education process to be held ransom by departments as it is in some institutions at the present time. If the chairs of departments are too dominant, then there must be a change in the administrative structure to diminish that influence.

4. The biggest challenge that we face in medical education is, how do we inculcate the knowledge, skills, attitudes and behaviors that are required to be a physician in a more effective, efficient and pleasant way than we do now? Does technology hold some promise for this in the future?

C.   James B. Erdmann, Ph.D. — "The Ecology of Curriculum Change"

I enjoyed reading Dr. Erdmann's manuscript very much. I am concerned, however, that it is too "discouraging" in tone and could lead a reader to believe that the reform should not be initiated. In fact, as I know Dr. Erdmann believes, curriculum change should be the most exciting development in a school of medicine since its impacts on all people who are part of that school and every single individual feels that they are an expert in this area. Dr. Erdmann's approach to the situation of defining the problem, defining the change, and reviewing the impact is very important. However, again, too much emphasis on problems of change could deter change even if the problems are well known to all. Certainly, some of the questions which Dr. Erdmann has listed would be important considerations in the conference, as would some of the problems which he outlined and which I am certain he could expand on at great length.

D. Vic Neufeld, M.D. — "Some Thoughts on Curriculum Change in Medical Education"

This well-written, targeted and thought-provoking essay needs thorough analysis by all participants in the conference. I was heartened to see his emphasis that little change in the health status of our society has occurred in the last decade even though the costs have steadily risen. I was puzzled, however, by the definition of "health" he was using and by his statement that some interventions used by physicians "do more harm than good." This certainly is worth exploring, since if, indeed, that thesis is defensible, it should be possible to analyze why that is true and to make educational changes designed to correct it.

I was very attracted to his enunciating of the system of faculty incentives and rewards but I doubt very much whether or not these have gone far enough. We must address what it is that brings pride, honor, dignity, and influence to a medical school by an individual faculty member and then determine how one makes these available to a person who spends the majority of his or her professional life involved in the educational process.

With regard to the accreditation process, I think we could well spend a considerable amount of time discussing that process and its impact on curricular change. The fundamental issues at stake are whether or not the accreditation process is designed to accredit a program leading to the M.D. degree, or is it designed to accredit a medical school. If it is the former, who is going to accredit the school? If it is the latter, does that give sufficient emphasis to the educational program? I certainly agree with the author's statement relative to "the intended end product."

With regard to licensure, this is a very thorny issue. While there is a common desire to have a single method of licensure, this is very difficult to achieve. Some individuals have suggested that all licensure occur as a result of an examination of an objective nature so there is no room for subjectivity or influence by the individuals who review the results. I, for one, do not agree that the National Board of Medical Examiners' test results are "abused," since I have always looked upon them as a tool to compare the performance of students at a single school with national norms. If one wishes to remove the NBME, then I think one must suggest alternatives to this mechanism of licensure.

The crux of the paper for this reviewer was the emphasis that "learning is an individual affair." As such, we must also conclude that learners learn in a variety of ways and that the way they learn varies from time to time and changes as they proceed through their professional and personal life. I am also pleased to see the author point out that role models are the most powerful influence—both good and bad.

E. Parker Small, M.D., et al. — "Possible Approaches for Improving Medical Education

This particular manuscript is very intriguing and quite challenging. Their suggestions relative to a reward system are, indeed, revolutionary and will be thought provoking. It is a novel idea in the United States, although it still exists in Switzerland in a sense where professors give all of the lectures because their salaries are tied to the number of lectures they give. I can assure you that this is a strong motivational factor in their showing and preparing for the lectures.

I agree with the authors' steps in effecting change except I
believe the first step in the process is the definition of the
problem. Based on that definition, one can answer the question, "Why is a change necessary?" Without definition of the
problems it is impossible to answer that question. Then comes
defining solutions to the problems including the goals of the
change, the format for implementation, and administrative
and resource changes to implement the change and an evaluation to determine whether the original goals had been met.
Why, in so many essays, is there such an overemphasis on
basic science education? In this area, we are already extracting the maximum possible out of the educational time available. I have often wondered why so little focus, attention, and
critical analysis is given to the clerkship phase of the undergraduate medical curriculum and on the "vacation" fourth
year. In these two areas there are gigantic blocks of educational time which, in my opinion, are inconsistently used, in-
adequately planned, poorly presented, and only briefly, if at
all, evaluated. Any one who spent any time on a clerkship
knows that the quality of instruction varies considerably depending upon the resident or attending who are involved and
the overall administration of the educational experience. It
would be very helpful to spend some time discussing how one
might effect curriculum change in this area since, as so often
happens, major change is implemented in the basic sciences
with a plan to continue the process sequentially into the clinical areas. Unfortunately, the process never reaches the clinical
areas.

I am also puzzled by the authors' suggestion that we need
to increase the contact in the basic sciences between faculty
and the students—to get back to where we were before. Yet, at
the same time, the authors propose that the time allocated for
instruction of the basic sciences be reduced to one-fourth of
that which now exists. If the laboratories in basic sciences of
the past twenty years did nothing else, they "protected" the
students from the faculty. They gave the students time to allow for a "settling" of the information they had been exposed
to, provided the students the opportunity to get to know each
other, to develop their interpersonal skills and to have some
fun. In addition, the laboratories allowed the development of

a sense of belonging which was built upon a close faculty-student relationship. Nowhere is this better exemplified than in the gross anatomy laboratories of the medical schools. The question is, "How to restore and/or recover this experience?" Is there another way to achieve it except by reestablishing laboratories? This seems to be a critical question if the goals of the curriculum are to be more than the acquisition of information and the sterile, inhuman application of that information in a clinical setting.

F. Reed G. Williams, Ph.D. — "How to Begin Reforming the Curriculum"

Dr. Williams' very fine manuscript brings out a number of perspectives which I think are of special significance and should be highlighted in the upcoming conference.

The first of these is that for an individual to become a physician, they require *practice* of the things which they are taught. Dr. Williams' discussion of this component of learning is exceedingly well done, as it represents something which I think many educators fail to appreciate.

Secondly, his enunciation of the fact that while clerkships provide opportunities to practice the skills and knowledge, it is rare when experts in the form of attending faculty members observe the process from start to finish, critiquing what they have seen and maximizing the educational experience. As such, the evaluation of student performances is certainly not carried out in a commendable way.

I also was attracted to his concept of a two-tiered level of evaluation of competency, including a "quick and dirty" assessment followed by a more indepth analysis. This, together with the diagnostic laboratory for clinical performance problem, is an excellent idea. In short, I enjoyed reading this manuscript and will look forward to discussing components of it at the conference.

G. "A New Pathway to General Medical Education at Harvard Medical School: The Oliver Wendell Holmes Society"

I enjoyed reviewing the information contained in the new proposed pathway at Harvard Medical School. It is interesting that only a small cohort of students will be selected to participate; that the educational experience will bridge from the premedical area to the first year of residency training; that a cohort of faculty will be assigned the responsibility of conducting this program; that social and academic prestige will be attached to it via a new society (The Oliver Wendell Holmes Society); that the educational experience will be "graduate-like" in the sense of small group tutorials, independent learning, computers, etc.; and that it will be financed by external sources.

Some concerns:

1. How will the program be financed once the experiment has been completed? Will this impact on its continuity?

2. How will this program be evaluated? The narrative suggests that evaluation is very important, but there are no specifics on how that is going to be achieved.

3. Given the smallness of the group and the close interaction between faculty and students, what arrangements are being made for the continued growth and development of the faculty who are involved in this undertaking? Will the rigid requirements for scientific productivity be applied to these faculty members in a manner similar to those who are involved in the usual activities of Harvard Medical School? Furthermore, what administrative change is being made to accommodate people who want to participate in this exciting venture?

4. Why is there not a greater emphasis on non-cognitive development of students including the proper values, attitudes, behaviors, etc.? This would seem an ideal opportunity to test different hypotheses in this arena.

While I recognize that this is a preliminary proposal and that it will not be activated until Fall of 1985, I would, on the one hand commend them for undertaking this assessment and coming up with this plan but at the same time would caution them about being certain that the evaluation of what they are trying is in place before they embark. I would also caution them to look carefully after the welfare of the faculty and students who are committing a portion of their career to this undertaking.

As an aside, I would commend them for including the requirement of a thesis. I think every medical school student should be required to prepare a thesis as a part of the graduation requirements.

II. Summary Thoughts

Based upon a review of the materials which I have received, some issues which emerge have received either too little emphasis or required greater emphasis than I see in the papers. These include the following:

A. Some attention must be given to the continuum of education. The Harvard proposal comes closest to this. Anything we do at the undergraduate level must be considered in the context of the larger continuum of medical education.

B. Some considerable discussion should be given to the reward system for faculty and the appropriate administrative structure to "house" people who are willing to invest their careers in the educational process.

C. I think it would be useful to discuss the kinds of people we are recruiting as faculty members. Are they generalists or are they specialists? It follows then, how should we structure a school of medicine to accomplish either the generalist or specialist functions so that medical education does not become a byproduct of the institutions called medical schools.

D. I think we should give some attention to public attitudes that exist now concerning physicians, the profession, and the health care delivery industry in general. A reflection of the public attitudes can be found in universities in the non-medical school areas and especially in places like nursing, law, mathematics, philosophy, etc. These attitudes within the universities, mirroring those on the outside, are shaping the destiny of medical school to a greater degree than any of us are willing to admit.

E. The new technologies including computers, automated libraries, etc., should be explored in some depth as should the biological revolution that is occurring. Only in the Harvard paper do I find a reference to the biological revolution, which I believe is going to dwarf significantly any revolution that has occurred in medicine in the history of mankind. It will, in my opinion, markedly alter, in fact revolutionize, our thinking about health and disease. Indeed, if we are talking about strategies for curricular change, we ought to be talking in the light of what we think will be in place from the new biology by the year 2010 and how we must prepare our students to participate/adjust to these changes.

F. If we are considering change, how do we maximize the learning from the changes which have already gone before? Too often there is change for changes sake with little attempt to learn what has been discovered and experienced before.

G. Possibly one of the strategies we might consider for curricular change is to use a "zero-base budget" philosophy. This would leave resource allocation, rewards, the organizational structure, etc., to follow the design of the educational program and not to serve as barriers for considering change.

H. In any discussions, it might be helpful to begin by asking the question, "Why must we change?" and secondly, "Can we change if we want to?" If we cannot answer the first question clearly and cannot answer the second question affirmatively, then the process should not proceed beyond that point.

I. We must be cognizant of external forces which may be available to assist in making change possible. Federal initiatives of the 1970's led to primary care training, including the family medicine movement, an increased emphasis on minority recruitment, the inculcation of certain subject matters into the curriculum, etc. This certainly is an external force which could be used to initiate change if, indeed, we think it is desirable.

J. Throughout these papers, there was very little discussion of quality. In my opinion, quality is the hallmark of the profession and the only thing, in the final analysis, that we can and must defend. Hence, I would like to see some discussion on that matter.

K. The extraordinarily critical importance of role models cannot be overemphasized. These individuals who serve as role models probably have more impact on an individual's growth and development by virtue of their impact on the individual's attitude, than all of the other things we do combined. How to select, develop and reward role models is, therefore, a critical element of initiating change in curriculum.

L. Finally, I would like to see a discussion on non-cognitive development. It appears, at this point in my evolving career, that the non-cognitive side of physicians' development may be infinitely more critical to the quality of care that they provide than all of the facts, skills, and principles that we attempt to force into their being. Further discussion of this thesis, therefore, might be useful.

March 1984

Alton I. Sutnick, M.D.

This is a propitious time for reform in medical education. As the relative reduction in federal research support has stimulated medical school faculties' efforts in other directions, and the complexities of reimbursement for professional services have mounted, members of medical school faculties are directing their efforts towards the educational missions of their institutions. Much of the interest appears to be centered upon structural changes in the curriculum. This response will comment on several threads of common interest that appear in the set of papers regarding curricular reform.

It is preferable for the curriculum to have some degree of flexibility to allow for modifications from time to time. Even adding an innovative course or two can be a valuable revision, and certainly an emphasis throughout the curriculum on issues such as geriatrics, continuing care, human values in medicine, socioeconomic factors in health care, etc. can provide a different perspective for the student. Such changes can be incorporated without requiring a major overhauling of the curriculum and may be addressed while building on the project on *General Professional Education of the Physician,* as suggested by Erdmann.

A mechanism should be introduced in each medical school for the identification of problems in the curriculum on an ongoing basis. We should always strive to upgrade the curriculum in our own individual way in keeping with the needs of a quality

180

medical education. It is generally agreed that continual attention to the educational process requires, as Neufeld says, a corporate sense that transcends departmental structure.

If the goals of medical education are defined in each medical school, there will be many constants, but there can be elements of variation among them. These differences might arise from factors such as the degree of emphasis on the arts and humanities, the attempt to address changing societal needs in the curriculum, or the degree to which faculty efforts are involved.

Reform often precipitates conservative reaction, as pointed out by Abrahamson. However, the potential excitement of innovation in medical education, together with a reduction in the sources of research funding, might be responsible for the devotion of more effort of our faculties to changes in educational techniques and curriculum design. It is important to recognize the concerns of faculty members who resist change. By addressing their needs, academic leaders may be able to involve them gradually in the process.

There are numerous differences in various approaches to curricular redesign and reorganization. This suggests that the medical schools are on the verge of even greater diversity of curricular design thus offering more distinct choices to their applicants.

Rationale for Curricular Reform

Changes in the curriculum should respond to educational needs and not be instituted for the sake of change itself. Consequently, problems existing in the curriculum must be identified before the solutions are designed.

External Factors

In changing the content of the medical school curriculum, educators should consider: 1) pressing national health needs, 2) new developments in scientific and clinical fields, and 3) the existing level of the students' knowledge as determined by internal and external means.

There are a number of factors that have impacted on the content of the medical curriculum in recent years. The government has exerted a major influence on the directions taken by medical education in a number of ways. It has fostered the development of family medicine as a medical specialty; encouraged the establishment of emergency medicine as a new discipline; and promoted new developments in training in primary care fields. Once responsible for the major growth of new and existing medical schools, government has now become an instrument of reduction in enrollment, cost containment and retrenchment. By withdrawal of support to medical education as a national resource, it has indirectly been responsible for the continuing escalation of medical school tuitions and fees, and the increasing parsimony in program development.

Demographic changes must also be considered in the development of curricula, with the continual graying of the U.S. population as a stimulus for the development of education programs in geriatrics. Geriatrics has in some ways developed from primary care training, to include comprehensiveness and continuity of care, accessibility of health care facilities and accountability for service. There is an emphasis on extended care, long-term care, home care, and the social issues involved in meeting the health needs of an elderly population. The change in pattern of disease in society together with the increase in the geriatric age group has resulted in a further emphasis on chronic diseases, nutrition and other preventive health measures.

This is an example of the impact of national health concerns on the undergraduate medical education curriculum. A curriculum should be able to respond flexibly to change, so that changing health needs of society do not result in obsolescence of the curriculum. A curriculum should be a dynamic mechanism for the interaction between clinical and basic science, which prepares the student for a lifetime of learning, rather than a rigid formulation that suits the needs of the moment.

In the context of developing major curricular revisions, organizational elements related to medical education should be considered, e.g. the standards of the Liaison Committee on Medical Education, the requirements of the National Residency Matching Program, the AAMC initiatives in the *General Professional Education of the Physician,* and AMA's *Future Directions in Medical Education.*

Impact of Curricular Changes on Departmental Structure

Some of the suggested new approaches to curricular development are proceeding along lines that differ from the traditional organization of medical schools. This may be a necessary route for innovation, but as indicated by Abrahamson, it can contribute to institutional problems when the innovation clashes with the existing institutional structure. It is difficult to develop curricular organization across departmental lines when the responsibility for promotions, salary increases, etc. lies with the department. It is much more convenient, and less costly for each course to be supervised by an individual department chairman, without the need to appoint new course directors. The faculty of each department expect to provide their teaching services within that department. Teaching in a program outside of that department may be perceived as an extra responsibility. Coordination of interdepartmental courses may require additional staff making it more costly than direct departmental teaching.

The traditional strength of medical school departments leads to another consideration in developing interdisciplinary courses; they may be seen as threats to departmental autonomy. Consequently, strong leadership is required to maintain the necessary communication and close cooperation between departments.

The development of interdisciplinary courses has the potential to lead to a consolidation of departments with, for example, the formation of a single Department of Physiology/Biochemistry, or a Department of Neuroscience. This may even be the first step to a practical approach to medical school organization related to the curriculum.

New approaches to medical care might be another impetus to spawn new departments via the establishment of new specialties. For example, some schools have established departments of emergency medicine, genetics, or geriatrics. Such departmental restructuring requires specific leadership activities of senior members of the faculty, and must be consistent with the requirements of graduate medical education programs.

Content

The content of the curriculum must be reviewed periodically. Changes in reimbursement mechanisms and new approaches to the organization of health care mandate that medical students be provided with a background in the economics of health care as well as an exposure to the forces that impact on the development of public health policy at the national, state, and local levels. Some aspects of the management of health care facilities including hospitals, free-standing ambulatory care facilities, ambulatory surgery centers, health maintenance organizations, preferred provider organizations, and other types of entities should be incorporated. The opportunities are always available to be innovative in the organization of the curriculum, and the introduction of new content. In recent years new emphases have been placed on emergency medicine, geriatrics, oncology, sexual dysfunction, social needs of patients, and even the inclusion of the arts and humanities in medical education.

The Student

It is generally agreed that there are substantial defects in an educational system that involves simply passive transmission of facts, emphasized by Erdmann and Williams. Learning has to be an active process, whether it involves laboratory work, small group discussions or interaction with surrogate patients. This must be recognized in any curriculum revision. It is necessary to incorporate an adequate evaluation process and some mechanism of direct observation of the student's clinical competence. Concern about the inadequacies of a multiple-choice examination as the sole evaluation mechanism are shared by most of the authors. Remediation should be available for all students in whom the need is identified. The complete course of instruction must be adequately mastered by every recipient of the M.D. degree.

A close relationship should be fostered between the faculty and students to expedite learning and increase the students' enthusiasm for their educational experience. It may also be helpful in the evaluation of the student.

The Faculty

Of course the faculty has the responsibility for undertaking curriculum reform under the leadership of the dean's office. I prefer to appoint a task force to initiate the process rather than to convene a large faculty retreat. A report of this task force would serve as the basis for discussion by the entire faculty, perhaps divided into a number of working groups.

I agree with Barrows that these educational changes will have little impact if medical school teachers are not adequately trained. Currently, there is a lack of programs and design strategies for the efficient and effective training of the faculty in educational technology and teaching effectiveness. Improvements in this link of the educational chain should be developed concurrently with the new curriculum directions.

Teaching is not adequately recognized and rewarded as a skill of the medical school faculty during a period of time when competition relates to research productivity and clinical competence. The department chairman can demonstrate financial gain to the department and frequently to the faculty member from research grants and patient fees, but value as a teacher is not reflected in incentive supplements or increasing departmental reserves. Both Neufeld and Barrows emphasize that it will become more and more essential for teaching skills to be considered as a major factor in the reward system for medical school faculty and academic departments.

April 1984

Appendix C:
Summary of Key Ideas Expressed in Protagonist and Reactor Papers

A. INSTITUTIONAL CHANGE

Factors Which Facilitate	Factors Which Impede

Abrahamson

- Reformers need to know the system.
- Anticipate problems and resistance.
- Modify the organization for the innovation.
- Obtain administrative support.
- All parties must feel involved.
- Changes must be consistent with the value system.
- Change must be perceived as valuable and challenging.
- There must be empathy for those who oppose change. "Whatever the *content* of the reformation, the *process* should reflect our best understanding of the dynamics of institutional change."

- "Natural" resistance to change.
- Vested interests.
- Self-serving power structure.
- Xenophobia.
- Institutional structures already in place.
- "Domino theory," i.e., "they want to change everything."
- "Guilt by association" — "reformers are kooks."

Barrows

- Develop a corporate response for education that crosses departments.
- Change administrative lines in education to facilitate the corporate response.

- Traditional values, rewards and expectations, as well as satisfaction with the way things are. Successful schools seem successful by the criteria and measurements usually employed, i.e., research scholars and NBME scores.

Brown

- Energize dean and faculty. Explain content of change. Justify it.
- Define the kind of physician we wish to produce, such that it can be measured.
- Change agent must understand the environment: level or declining resources, faculties run the schools, environments from which our students come, faculty are not conservative in their research.

Factors Which Facilitate	Factors Which Impede

Dignam
- Alter the distinction between basic science and clinical medicine.
- Provide problem-based instruction, without lectures.
- Persuade departments to be more responsible for the overall performance of their students.

Erdmann
- Improve organization of courses (but this requires extra effort).
- Introduce problem-based small group— to increase self-motivated learning and provide relevance to learning.
- Reform assessment methods to make them more relevant to curricular aims (but this may be seen to reduce objectivity of assessment and will require extra effort).

• Loss of objectivity of assessment and extra effort following from use of assessment reform.
• Extra effort required by staff.

Gibbs
- Involve faculty (and administrators) in review process before attempting change.
- Develop better ways to document faculty teaching efforts.

Heins
- Challenge each department to: 1) remove unnecessary content; 2) provide small group learning; 3) introduce problem-solving exercises; 4) modify examinations to measure thinking and problem-solving; 5) foster self-learning; 6) utilize computer technology.

Moy
- Key off the pride of the institution in educational excellence.
- Provide an authoritative voice, probably the dean, external or internal to the school, that can be properly orchestrated to encourage change.
- Provide permission for experimentation in education by the faculty.

Factors Which Facilitate   **Factors Which Impede**

Moy

- Allow the school to realize or admit that their primary concern is educating students, that they are an educational institution.
- Key off national discontent as provided by the AAMC-GPEP activities; provide a "non-permission" for status quo.
- LCME essential to create better expectations.
- Involve the students in policy development as they are the recipients of educational excellence.
- Publicize such events as the New Pathway, an innovative, appropriate curricular change undertaken by a well-recognized traditional university as a stimulus to other schools.

Neufeld

- Major initiatives are needed to strengthen research (and development) in medical education.
- Develop informal networks of institutions with similar interests in medical education for producing materials, reports, etc.
- A cadre of educational leaders—a few individuals who make the educational program their primary task.
- A system of faculty incentives and rewards. Essential elements include: 1) recognition that there are various educational roles; 2) promotion and tenure statements that educational contributions are recognized as essential.
- A quantitative record of an individual's contribution to education.
- Orientation to the curriculum for new faculty.
- A corporate sense; it is critical that the "community of scholars" in a medical school has a sense of the relative priorities of institutional goals.

Factors Which Facilitate	**Factors Which Impede**

Neufeld
- A statement of educational purpose—primarily a description of the "end product" which the medical curriculum is designed to produce.
- A long-range view, with educational leadership that is clear and firm about long-range timing and methods to achieve them.
- Medical schools should propose a change in the accreditation process so that institutional self-study addresses: 1) What is intended end-product? 2) What evidence you are producing this product, 3) Are teaching/learning processes arranged to facilitate/achieve this? 4) Do students enjoy their medical education?

Robbins
- Changes derived from external pressure. For example, government may cause changes by backing up its request with resouces in order to achieve the stated purpose or make access to certain resources contingent upon compliance (e.g. "financial carrot" system).
- Dissatisfaction of student and faculty with traditional teaching programs.
- Structure changes so that curriculum matters and changes involve faculty and students.
- Accrediting bodies.
- Dean committed to changes.
- Young chairmen eager to experiment new ideas.
- Foundation grants to support planning and implementation.

Factors Which Impede (Robbins):
- Hospital organization set up more for service than teaching, and to compete for students' attention.

Russe
- Common perception of need as reflected in GPEP. Strategy for change must be carefully contemplated. Must make curriculum an institutional rather than a departmental matter.

Factors Which Impede (Russe):
- Change can create martyrs. Difficult to accomplish. Perception of lectures as the "path of righteousness."

| **Factors Which Facilitate** | **Factors Which Impede** |

Schwarz

- Must define reason for change in language all parties will understand.
- Must be some benefit for all parties, whether money, pride, or FTE's, etc. (reward system).
- Change needs a small cadre of revolutionaries. Change must go from the top (instition, administration) on down.
- The institution accreditation process must give sufficient import to educational matters (in comparison to research activities, etc.).
- Must have an evaluation system in place for change before embarking.
- Decreasing public confidence in the medical profession.
- Zero-based budgeting.
- External incentives, e.g., the federal government.

- Big units will conspire to take resources, power, etc. from small.
- Must decrease departmental power over curriculum in favor of institutional approach.

Small

- Establish national network (led by SIU) for use of simulated patient/practical instructor in the teaching of history-taking and physical exam.
- In workshop, have faculty and students develop a plan to improve the educational program, including adequate feedback and rewards to assume that system evolves toward attainment of goals.
- Determine faculty and student perception of how well goals are being met.
- Have workshop for faculty and students to exchange views of problems in medical education.
- Have faculty agree on goals.

Sutnick

- Relative reduction in federal research support plus complexities of reimbursement for professional services may stimulate faculty's efforts to other matters (e.g. education).

- Difficult to develop inter-departmental curricular changes when promotion, salary increases lie within department.

Factors Which Facilitate	**Factors Which Impede**

Sutnick

- Mechanism to identify problems in curriculum.
- Provide a "corporate sense that transcends departmental structure."
- Governmental pressure (grants for family medicine, cost containment).
- Standards of LCME: requirements by NRMP: AAMC's GPEP; AMA's *Future Directions in Medical Education.*
- Appoint task force to initiate process, rather than convene a large faculty retreat.
- Reward teaching.
- Dynamic mechanism between basic and clinical science.

Williams

- Adopt financial structure which holds faculty accountable for quality teaching and rewards them directly.

Factors Which Impede

- Recognize concerns of faculty members who resist change. By addressing their needs, academic leaders may be able to involve them gradually in the process.

B. INDIVIDUAL CHANGE

Factors Which Facilitate	Factors Which Impede

Abrahamson

- Complacency.
- Habit.
- "But it worked for us before."
- Selective perception.
- Ego involvement with status quo.

Barrows
- Encourage recognition and reward for scholarship and excellence in education.
- Provide promotion, pay, status and perquisites for educational endeavor and scholarship.
- Make sure that the individual departments, members and chairmen, respect and value a member that devotes a large amount of time to educational scholarship.
- Improve faculty knowledge and skills in the area of education and educational science through a variety of experiences, workshops, fellowships, apprenticeships.

Brown

Dignam
- Train teachers to teach.

Erdmann

- Anxieties by both students and staff about problem-based learning.

Factors Which Facilitate	Factors Which Impede

Gibbs

Heins
- Money.
- National Teaching Award to be given at the AAMC meetings; awards for teaching within each medical school.

- Difficulty in obtaining research dollars, necessitating increased concentration on writing more research applications and doing more research.
- Increased efforts by faculty to deal with cost containment.
- Increased competition for patients as a distraction.
- Increasing faculty stress.

Moy
- Key off the pride of the individual faculty person for excellence in education and the value of the product produced by his or her school.
- Change the system to reward scholarly work in education.

Neufeld

Robbins

- Personal incentives of the faculty are not emphasized.
- Financial incentives are not directed towards teaching nor is peer approbation oriented in this way. Recognition is often based on research, publication and practice.
- While teaching cannot be judged in quantitative terms, research, publication and practice can.

Russe
- Need for faculty recognition and development of appropriate incentives in curricular change. Need appropriate reward system for good teachers.

Factors Which Facilitate

Factors Which Impede

Schwarz

- Faculty must be challenged to take scholarly, experimental approach to educational matters.
- Possibly separate "science-oriented" faculty into different organizational structures, allowing different reward systems.
- Must be a reward system for people devoted to the educational process.

- Cries of academic freedom.
- Traditional lack of reward system for educational efforts.

Small

- Students and faculty must get to know each other well enough so that faculty can directly observe students' growth.
- Give each class of students a substantial amount of dollars to divide as students see fit among their teachers.
- Give course directors a substantial amount of dollars to divide as they see fit among their teachers.

- Lack of feedback and rewards for good teaching, particularly in competition with direct feedback and rewards for other faculty roles.
- Lack of communication between students and faculty.

Sutnick

- Strong leadership in department would allow necessary communication and close cooperation between departments.
- Provide efficient and effective training of faculty in educational technology and teaching effectiveness.

Williams

- Students do the learning.
- Provide for learning in a functional context.
- Provide early and multiple opportunities to practice: practical instructors, practical exercises, and standardized/simulated patients.
- Provide feedback from peers and faculty.
- Observe experts and other students work up same patient.

C. TESTING

Abrahamson

Barrows

Brown
- Few of us regard the NBMEs or any other test as adequate to measure the qualities of the physician we wish to produce.
- How do we measure the physician? The answer to that defines the curriculum and makes the process of reform obvious.

Dignam

Erdmann
- Abolition of MCQs is likely to be helpful, but their replacement by other means may cause worries about objectivity.

Gibbs
- Best stimulus to active learning behavior is modification of our evaluation system.

Heins

Moy

Neufeld
- Rather than scapegoat the NBME, join with the agency to accelerate development of appropriate evaluation tools.

Robbins

Russe
- Students required to pass criterion-based certifying examination on each "subject" in the pre-clinical curriculum.
- Student progress during pre-clinical curriculum measured by performance on criterion-referenced examinations and performance in small group problem-solving sessions.
- Promotion to year 3 requires passage of (a) all criterion-referenced examinations; (b) measures of clinical reasoning, history taking, physical diagnosis, interpersonal skills; and (c) NBME-Part I.

Schwarz

- NBME use is okay, since it provides an objective, cross-institutional standard. Those wanting to eliminate must propose an alternative.
- Need constant observation by faculty of students applying knowledge, doing professional things, etc., to improve assessment.
- Need two-tiered evaluation of competency: "quick and dirty," followed by in-depth assessment methods (a la Williams).
- Graduation requirements should include a thesis.

Small

- NBME Parts I and II test only fact recognition. Time per MCQ must be increased so that higher cognitive functions can be tested. Implies reducing total number of MCQs. Implies that applicants' scores be not by discipline but only for basic and clinical sciences.
- Urgent NBME charge is experimentation with non-MCQ formats. Simulated patients and patient evaluators seem exciting possibilities.
- In medical school, the triple jump exam should be used to evaluate data base, data management and data acquisition.
- In medical schools, clinical evaluation should involve simulated patient/ practical instructors.
- A review of microbiology final exams in 24 schools and the NBME test item library shows 90% of MCQs test isolated fact recognition. This leads students to pursue quick answers instead of investigative processes, to blindly accept faculty's word rather than develop critical analysis skills.

Sutnick

- Incorporate an adequate evaluation process and some mechanism of direct observation of the student's clinical competence.
- Concerns about the inadequacies of multiple-choice exams.

Williams

- Diagnostic tests which help to discriminate deficiencies and from which appropriate remedial activities can be identified and retested.

D. STUDENT OBJECTIVES FOR HEALTH CARE

Abrahamson

Barrows

Brown

Dignam
- More self-education.
- Relocation of basic science time throughout the courses.
- Problem-based learning.

Erdmann

Gibbs

Heins

Moy

Neufeld
- Related to the price-competitive environment; medical schools need to anticipate in the curricular changes needed to produce physicians who can provide leadership in private health care systems.

Robbins

Russe
- Reasoning and problem-solving as opposed to rote learning.
- Ability to use current medical literature.
- Use of the computer as "memory extender, consulting knowledge system and decision aid."
- Critical attitude toward "given truths."
- Habits of life-long learning.

Schwarz
- Role models are critical in influencing students, good or bad.
- Must focus on "non-cognitive" objectives such as "proper values, attitudes and behaviors," as well as cognitive things.

Small
- Apply problem-solving skills, data acquisition and analysis to pathophysiologic processes taking place in their patients.

Sutnick
- Geriatrics.
- Economics of health care.
- Exposure to the forces that affect the development of public health policy at the national, state and local levels.
- Management of health care facilities.
- A complete course of instruction must be adequately mastered by every recipient of the M.D. program.

Williams
- Make appropriate discriminations.
- Perform technical skills appropriately.
- Reason effectively.
- Coordinate knowledge, reasoning ability, interpersonal skills and technical skills.

E. SUGGESTIONS FOR CURRICULAR REFORM

Abrahamson
- Whatever the *content* of the reformation, the *process* should reflect our best understanding of the dynamics of institutional change.

Barrows
- A faculty retreat to assign priorities to the various activities of the medical school, hopefully attaching the highest priority to young men and women to be physicians. Also, at such a retreat the competencies expected of their product should be described. Hopefully, this will include such things as critical thinking, ability to problem-solve, self-directed study skills, appreciation of the whole patient, etc.
- Educate the teaching faculty.
- Develop corporate responsibility for educational activities (as above).
- Provide rewards for teaching (as above).
- Develop accurate, relevant assessment tools to provide accurate feedback about student progress.

Brown

Dignam
- Fewer lectures.

Erdmann
- Course reorganization to increase efficiency.
- Small group teaching.
- Assessment reform.

Gibbs

Heins
- Any change should be evaluated, particularly from the standpoint of the patient's satisfaction. Reintroduce meaningful lab experiences to provide small group interactions and increase basic science faculty contact and problem-solving.
- Introduce in the clinical years a system in which the attending interacts with students at the bedside, probably in small groups, as was the situation many years ago.

Moy

Neufeld

Robbins

Russe
- Need a balance between imparting information and instilling a spirit of perpetual learning.
- Students learn cognitive content of preclinical curriculum by independent individual and group study, assisted by "resource" faculty, clinical problems, and a syllabus prepared by faculty.
- A faculty "resource person" aids in: (a) definition of learning goals, (b) preparation of syllabi, (c) supplementary educational support, (d) coordination of learning resources.
- Students organized into small learning groups (8) with clinical facilitator who uses Socratic method.
- Focus of group activity is clinical problems (PBLM, simulations, real patients) chosen to emphasize curricular objectives, including basic science content and clinical reasoning.
- Lots of use of computers for learning/instruction, data base and file management, etc.

Schwarz
- Organ system approach may not be all bad, may be an evolutionary plateau.
- Put more emphasis on changing clerkships and 4th year "vacation" year than on preclinical years, where "we are already extracting maximum possible out of the educational time available."
- Better coordination and especially follow-through between basic science and clinical years.
- Need haven (from faculty) during initial years where students can settle-in, get to know each other, etc. Old "labs" served this purpose. Are there alternatives?
- Need settings for practice of professional skills with observation and feedback.
- Anticipate advances in the new biology by year 2010, and shape curriculum to these.

Small
- Do not attempt to involve all faculty in the regular curriculum. Those interested mostly in research and graduate education, involve only in special projects such as independent study projects.
- Condense basic sciences to one semester.
- Devote three-fourths of basic science time to solving clinical problems. Use variety of formats (PBLMs, POPs, CPCs), progressively more complex.

Sutnick
- Emphasize arts and humanities.
- Address changing societal needs in curriculum.
- Problems in curriculum must be identified first before solutions are designed.
- Curriculum changes should consider pressing national health needs, new scientific and clinical development, and existing level of students' knowledge as determined by internal and external means.
- Geriatrics program.
- Development of interdisciplinary courses leads to a consolidation of department.
- Learning has to be an active process, and remediation should be available for all students who need it.

Williams
- Minimum of 50% of the student's time in years 1 and 2 should be in practice of relevant discrimination, technical and interpersonal skills, clinical reasoning activities, and use of knowledge in clarifying and resolving patient problems.

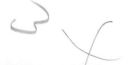